THE FEEL FULL DIET

THE
FEEL FULL
DIET

STEVEN R. PEIKIN, M.D.

Director, Jefferson Nutrition Program
Jefferson Medical College

Recipes and Menus by
Gloria Kaufer Greene

ATHENEUM　　*New York*　　1987

Library of Congress Cataloging in Publication Data

Peikin, Steven R.
  The feel-full diet.

  Includes index.
  1. Reducing diets.   2. Cholecystokinin.
  3. Appetite depressants.   I. Title.
RM222.2.P453   1987   613.2'5   86-47927
ISBN 0-689-11789-2

Published simultaneously in Canada by Collier Macmillan Canada, Inc.
Manufactured by Haddon Craftsmen, Scranton, Pennsylvania
Designed by Kathleen Carey
First Edition

FOR PHYLLIS AND DAVID,
good friends, the best of parents

7136721

ACKNOWLEDGMENTS

I would like to thank all the medical students, graduate students, postdoctoral fellows, and collaborators who have worked with me in my gastrointestinal hormone laboratory at Jefferson Medical College. Each piece of information they generated contributed to the conception of this book. Special thanks go to Robert Crochelt, Ph.D., and Carol McLaughlin, Ph.D. Morton Klein encouraged me to write this book. His continued efforts to bring nutritional information to the public are commendable.

I wish to express a special debt of gratitude to Cheryl Clifford, R.D., of the Jefferson Nutrition Program, for assistance with recipes and review of the manuscript, and David Rorvik of Proteus, Inc. for valuable help in the preparation of the manuscript. I have to thank Elenor Franco and Shirley Shelton for severe wear and tear on their minds and fingertips in the typing of the manuscript.

Finally, my wife, Lori Snodgrass, deserves my special gratitude not only for her unwavering support but also for her valuable contributions in Chapter 11 on Weight Maintenance and Chapter 12 on Exercise.

CONTENTS

ix

INTRODUCTION

How This Diet Differs from Others and What It Can Do for You That They Can't

THE "FEEL FULL" BREAKTHROUGH

If you are overweight, the reasons are most likely physical, *not* psychological. Simply recognizing this fact is a breakthrough in itself, for both science and society. And now that we are beginning to understand the biochemical basis of obesity, we can, at last, do something effective about it.

The diet described in this book uses important new discoveries related to the body's mechanisms for signaling "satiety," or fullness. One of these mechanisms involves the "hunger hormones." I and my colleagues have been investigating substances produced by the body that help signal fullness, hormones that tell the body, if everything is working properly, when to *stop* eating.

I know I don't have to tell most of you that things don't *always* work properly. Plenty of excess pounds attest to that. It is possible that at some point in the distant past all of these mechanisms did work effectively and that they have since been subverted by a variety of factors. In the high-technology, high-stress world of today, many of us tend to wolf down large quantities of food in short periods of time, overriding many of the satiety mechanisms I have been studying. Our lifestyle may be making it increasingly difficult for us to sense the signals that tell our brains and bodies when enough really *is* enough.

But don't despair. The mechanisms and the signals are still there. If you're having trouble "hearing" them, this book will help you rediscover them, and, more important, it will help you use them to your advantage *without* having to change radically *what* you eat. The "feel full" breakthrough alters the *way* you eat—but in a way most people find more pleasurable than restrictive.

PROVEN RESULTS

The Feel Full Diet is the centerpiece of the Jefferson Nutrition Program at Jefferson Medical College in Philadelphia. Hundreds of individuals have participated in this program with excellent results. Unlike most of the so-called "fad" diets, this one is being tested in a clinical hospital setting. Weight loss is adjusted in this diet to proceed at a prudent, healthy rate—two pounds per week on average (with an optional, accelerated program after the first four weeks, as will be explained in detail later in this book). The fact that this diet provides a feeling of fullness—something lacking in most diets—helps explain why the fall-off rate is so low. People don't quit this diet as they do most fad or crash diets because they get varied and tasty fare, a nutritionally balanced diet that does *not* leave them feeling hungry.

The Feel Full Diet produces a sense of fullness while keeping total caloric intake low. Some other diets have tried to increase the feeling of fullness by promoting very high fiber intake. For a variety of health reasons, almost all Americans could profit from increasing somewhat the amount of fiber in their overly refined diets. But eating very large amounts of high-fiber foods to stave off hunger requires substantial dietary change and can produce gastrointestinal distress, which, even if short term in some people, quickly discourages adherence to a new diet.

The Feel Full Diet does, in fact, encourage increased fiber intake, but the increase is moderate, and the diet does not depend on this factor for its ability to satisfy appetite. Far more important is a unique component of our diet—one we call "the satietizer" (say-she-ĕ-tizer). Satietizers have the opposite effect of appetizers, which are supposed to sharpen hunger. If properly prepared *and* if eaten at the right time in relation to the main course, these satietizers are actually "satisfiers." They help turn off your craving for high-calorie fats and proteins—help turn off hunger signals in general.

TAMING THE HUNGER HORMONES

Our discoveries related to hormones that switch hunger on and off provide something truly new in dieting. Several of these hormones are now under study. One that has been much in the news is the hormone cholecystokinin, a tongue twister I will henceforth refer to simply as CCK. I have been studying this hormone for many years and have published numerous scientific papers on its properties. CCK enters the bloodstream after a meal and stimulates the gallbladder and pancreas, which deposit bile and digestive enzymes in the intestines. CCK has another important function: it signals the brain that the person is full and thus helps terminate the meal. Much of what has been said about this substance in the popular press has been erroneous. Dietary manipulation through *timing* of food intake, among other things, is the only readily available way to modify the activity of the hunger hormones, such as CCK. At present there are no *effective* CCK pills.

I and various of my coworkers have demonstrated conclusively that certain hormones control satiety—fullness—in numerous animals and in humans. One of our most important findings is that many people who are obese are overweight for biochemical and *not* psychological reasons. For instance, I've found that one form of obesity is due almost entirely to insufficient numbers of various hormone receptors in the body. Without enough of these receptors the body can't adequately receive the signals that say it's time to stop eating.

One of the most gratifying results of finding biochemical rather than psychological causes of obesity has been seeing many of my patients shed guilt along with the pounds they've carried with them for so many years. The psychological effects of obesity can be even more devastating than the physical ones. The overweight person typically thinks he or she is somehow "bad" or lacking in willpower. Now our research is showing how mistaken and outdated this notion is. Medical science is demonstrating for the first time in any substantial way that obesity can have biochemical bases far more commonplace than ever before suspected. And fortunately, those biochemical defects that contribute to obesity are vulnerable to attack and correction.

WHY MOST OTHER DIETS FAIL

Most diets fail in the long run for one of two reasons: (1) they don't restrict calories sufficiently or (2) if they do adequately restrict calories, they don't suppress appetite. Diets that are generous with calories result in either no weight loss or in such slow weight loss that the dieter quickly loses interest and motivation. Most of the "fad" or "crash" diets, however, are actually too restrictive with calories. The typical "starvation" or "ketogenic" diet, providing fewer than 1000 calories per day, results in rapid weight loss, no doubt about it, but it leaves the dieter feeling famished, and soon he or she is reaching into the pantry for forbidden high-calorie goodies.

Worse, these crash diets are usually nutritionally unbalanced. There is growing evidence that they burn up more muscle and lean body mass than they do fat. Then, when the dieter gives up on the diet—the "fall-off" rate on most fad diets is eventually nearly 100 percent—the weight that is regained is mostly fat. The end result is a body composed of more fat than ever before. That is why it can now be said that many diets are actually fattening!

To get a diet to burn fat more selectively while sparing the lean body mass, it's important to provide ample, but not excessive, calories. It's also vital to make sure the diet is the "mixed" nutrient type, not one that has you stuffing down one—monotonous—type of food each day.

PREVIEW OF THE FEEL FULL DIET

The Feel Full Diet has the optimal number of calories and the right combination of nutrients to produce sufficient weight loss to sustain motivation. It is nutritionally balanced and does not in its basic form require vitamin/mineral supplementation. It provides for a wide variety of different foods and is never boring or bland. It minimizes the number of changes you have to make in the standard American way of eating, although it still manages to increase fiber and reduce fat. Beyond all this, however, the diet produces something entirely new: a way to induce a feeling of fullness *before* you have overeaten. Furthermore, the Feel Full Diet helps alter body metabolism in ways that encourage *long-term* weight loss.

I have found that, at present, there is virtually no way to prevent the desire to *start* eating. But because of our research and that of others, we do now have a way to *stop* eating before we've eaten too much. My diet is designed to allow the dieter to feel full after eating less than normal. To achieve this goal, the diet contains foods that stimulate release of the body's CCK, an antihunger hormone, and other related substances. And because the *rate* at which food is digested and reaches the hormone-containing cells in the small intestine is of crucial importance, *correct timing* of the courses of the meal is a vital part of the regimen.

The "satietizer," about which I'll have a lot more to say later in this book, is a small first course that sets the stage for earlier than normal "fullness." Next comes the intrameal interval, another unique feature of the Feel Full Diet. This is a twenty- or thirty-minute interlude between the first course (satietizer) and the main course. During this interval the dieter may not eat anything else (except water or diet beverage) but may move about, read, talk, work, and so on. Most of the dieters in our program at Jefferson enjoy this interval. And when they sit down to eat the main course they find they are not particularly hungry—or at least not nearly as hungry as usual. The satietizers themselves come in a wide variety—from convenience items to gourmet selections. They can be eaten while the rest of the meal is still being prepared or can even be eaten at one's office desk before going out to lunch. Many of them are highly portable and can be prepared in large batches at one time and frozen for future use.

You'll find recipes for many satietizers and sample meal plans in the second half of this book. These have been prepared by the noted food and nutrition journalist and cookbook author Gloria Kaufer Greene in collaboration with me, and have been reviewed by our registered dietitian, Cheryl Clifford.

The Feel Full Diet is *not* a crash diet. The basic program provides for 1200 to 1300 calories per day. This is a safe and effective program of caloric restriction that does not require a physician's supervision unless you have some particular health problem. Rate of weight loss, of course, depends upon the individual's height and initial weight and body build, but *average* weight loss on the diet is two pounds per week.

Once ideal weight is achieved—I'll show you how to determine what is "ideal" for you—I'll give you the information you'll need to determine how many calories you should consume to maintain that weight, again taking into account your individual characteristics and needs.

In addition to the basic regimen, the book will provide an optional program aimed predominantly at *highly motivated women* who want faster—yet still safe—results. This optional diet will never provide fewer than 1000 calories per day and *will* include specific vitamin/mineral supplementation. An optional program will also be provided for *men* who find 1300 calories per day *too restrictive*. This optional male diet will not exceed 1800 calories per day.

Yet another variation on the basic program incorporates *optional* exercise, with different caloric requirements. Some individuals are more likely than others to benefit from this diet/ exercise combination. I'll help you determine whether you are one of them. Exercise can be important in altering the metabolic "set point" that determines, in each individual, the weight that the body tries to maintain despite any effort at dieting. Manipulating the set point is, in itself, no substitute for diet but, in combination with diet, can be very useful for most individuals.

Now let's begin. In the first chapter you'll learn more about the exciting discoveries that make this unique new diet possible.

I

Putting the
Feel Full Diet
to Work *for You*

1

What Makes You Hungry?
What Makes You Full?
(*The Answers May Surprise You*)

CONCENTRATE ON STOPPING RATHER
THAN ON NOT STARTING

PEOPLE WHO READ about my research in the magazines and newspapers constantly write to me asking, "Doctor, why do I *always* feel hungry? Why, no matter how much I eat, do I *never* feel full? Why do I eat until I'm miserable? How can I kill this ravenous appetite?" There's a lot of genuine anguish in these letters and also a lot of true misunderstanding about just what it is that controls food intake. Before we learn in subsequent chapters how specific individuals have successfully dealt with both their anguish and their hunger, let's look at some of the basics on which the Feel Full Diet is built.

Many people, if they think about hunger and fullness at all,

3

typically do so along these lines: "I'm hungry when I haven't eaten. I'm full after I've eaten." Most of those people are lean and always have been. But, as plenty of you know, it isn't that simple for everybody. Some 34 million Americans are now significantly overweight. *They* know it is possible to eat—and eat a lot—and still not feel full. So they eat still more. Thus the old simplistic notions about hunger and fullness will no longer do —not if we really want to construct a diet that will work—one that will address the biochemical bases of obesity.

So let's dig a little deeper. There is no question that two separate sensations determine how much we eat. One of these sensations we call "hunger" or "appetite," which we describe as a desire to eat. The other sensation is "fullness" or "satiety," a feeling of satisfaction that induces us to stop eating. Both of these sensations, however, can become badly distorted. Hunger may be persistent, occur too often after eating, and so on. And the feeling of fullness that we rely upon to induce us to stop eating may actually be more like *pain* than pleasure in some people, as a result of overeating; in other words, it may arise too late.

But here, at least, we have a point at which to begin, and what I'm eventually going to demonstrate to you is that, contrary to the common wisdom, it's better to focus on stopping rather than on not starting. Here's what I mean. Despite years of research, we still know next to nothing about the control of appetite. In other words, we have no handle on how to prevent people from wanting to *start* eating. If you're hungry, you'll eat no matter what. Yet most diets and "diet aids" try to turn off hunger so that people won't start eating. And as most of you know, most diets and diet aids don't work. That's because there is no scientific basis for diets predicated on appetite control. We do, however, know quite a bit now about *fullness,* and this new knowledge provides the background for a diet based on the manipulation of the "satiety" (fullness) signals and mechanisms so that we can learn to *stop* eating before we've consumed too much.

Most diets—and therefore most dieters—have been barking up the wrong tree, one that so far hasn't borne any fruit. It's time to reorient ourselves away from the hunger signals and toward the fullness signals, where we actually have a good chance to do something effective.

The following discussion will help you better understand how hunger and fullness work in the normal course of events. And in the next chapter I'll show you how we discovered we could modify some of these events to assist many of those 34 million Americans in their battle with "girth control."

There are three phases that control food intake and digestion. It's important to understand a little about each of them.

THE BRAIN PHASE

Ultimately, the brain controls both hunger and fullness. Hunger begins when the so-called "feeding center" of the brain is activated by unknown stimulants. If you haven't eaten for a while, a sensation of hunger ensues, even if you can't see or smell food. If you *can* see or smell food, or are good at imagining it, this initial brain activation is further amplified. The brain sends signals to the stomach, pancreas, and intestines via the vagus nerve. These signals stimulate the acids of the stomach and the digestive enzymes of the pancreas. They also start the muscles of the intestines and stomach working, producing the familiar "growling" or "rumbling" we all associate with hunger pangs. All of this primes the system to receive food and to begin processing it immediately.

THE STOMACH PHASE

The stomach or gastric phase governing food intake is the first phase in which fullness mechanisms come into play. As the stomach fills up, its walls become distended or stretched. This distension triggers a new signal, again via the vagus nerve, to the brain. This signal goes to the "satiety" or fullness center, not to the feeding center of the brain. The signal says, in effect, that fullness is occurring. Even a balloon inserted into the stomach and then inflated, causing the stomach wall to stretch, can send a signal of fullness to the brain. Meanwhile, the presence of food in the stomach causes further acid secretion and the release of various other chemicals that aid in digestion.

THE INTESTINAL PHASE

In this phase food begins to pass from the stomach into the small intestine. As soon as protein and fat begin to enter the small intestine they trigger the release of CCK, the hormone I mentioned in the Introduction. We and others have shown that CCK is a naturally occurring substance in the body that helps to control food intake by stimulating a further sensation of fullness just as urgent as that produced by gastric distension. CCK may, in fact, have direct effects on the stomach wall and the brain itself (interestingly, we find as much CCK in the brain as we do in the small intestine). In any event, we know that CCK plays a role in gastric distension, resulting in fullness signals to the brain.

The release of CCK and other substances during this phase stimulates the gallbladder and pancreas, both of which are active in the digestive process. Food passing from the stomach into the small intestine also causes release of a variety of substances, which ultimately turn off the gastric phase of digestion.

The intestinal phase is, by far, the most important for both digestion and the sensation of fullness. You can sever the vagus nerve—the main communication link between the brain and the stomach—and digestion will still occur. (This operation is often performed in the treatment of peptic ulcer disease and has no major adverse effect on digestion.) You can eliminate the gastric phase by removing the stomach (as is sometimes done to treat cancers of the stomach) and, again, digestion proceeds very nicely in the small intestine. Try to remove the intestinal phase, though, and you're in real trouble. If the small intestine is inoperative, death from malnutrition is inevitable without intravenous feeding.

The intestinal phase is similarly dominant when it comes to signaling fullness. We now know that even with the vagus nerve severed (putting the stomach out of touch with the brain), a sensation of fullness can still occur. The classic experiment that demonstrated the importance of the intestinal phase of fullness was performed by Dr. Gerald Smith at Cornell University Department of Psychology. He operatively placed a tube in the stomach and another in the small intestine of a rat. Both tubes exited outside the abdomen. If the stomach tube was left open, everything the rat ate (it was fed liquid meals only) immediately drained into a pan at the bottom of the cage. In this instance there was, of course, no filling of the stomach and thus no distension of the stomach walls. Nor was there any entrance of food into the small intestine below the stomach. In this case, the rat ate nonstop!

But when just a *small* amount of the liquid meal that had drained into the pan was injected into the small intestine the rat quickly stopped eating and exhibited the usual behavior (grooming, resting, and so forth) associated with fullness in that animal. Furthermore, the feeling of fullness occurred even though there was no distension of the stomach. It has also been shown that the same result can be achieved *without* putting any food into the small intestine if CCK is injected into the bloodstream.

LOOKING AHEAD: LEARNING HOW TO TAKE ADVANTAGE OF THE INTESTINAL PHASE

Now that I've shown how important the small intestine is in signaling/sensing fullness, let me show you how most people never use the intestinal phase to their advantage. This matter will be explored in greater detail later, but I want to show you right now how all this technical information I'm asking you to familiarize yourselves with has a very practical purpose.

Here, briefly, is the gist of it: To activate the intestinal phase of fullness, food—and not necessarily very much food, as we've seen—has to pass from the stomach into the duodenum, the foremost portion of the small intestine. Food does not pass immediately from the stomach into the duodenum. This process takes time. In fact, for the stomach to empty completely may take four, five, or six hours after a large meal.

We have discovered, however, that within twenty or thirty minutes after eating, enough food gets into the duodenum to stimulate release of CCK. So what's the problem? you're asking. The problem is that the CCK fullness signals don't kick in until after most people have wiped their mouths, used the finger bowls, and patted their bellies after having already consumed a 1000 (or more)-calorie meal.

As you'll soon discover, the Feel Full Diet alters the way you eat so that the all-important intestinal phase of food intake/digestion has a chance to go to work for you.

In the next chapter you'll learn about some of the experiments we and others have done—experiments that led to and made possible the Feel Full Diet.

2

Harnessing the Feel Full Mechanisms

The Scientific Basis for the Feel Full Diet

IS THERE ANY REASON WHY *THIS*— OR *ANY*—DIET SHOULD WORK?

IT'S AMAZING HOW many people are willing to jump head-long into a new diet without first investigating whether there is any convincing evidence that the diet really does or should work. Most diets are utterly unsupported by any scientific evidence, clinical trials, or other testing. Most lack even any sound theoretical underpinnings. In brief, there is no proof that most diets work nor any compelling reason to believe that they should work, other than on a short-term basis.

9

The diet field has never been one to exhibit much concern for scientific method. In truth, both the self-proclaimed "diet experts" *and* the dieting public know this. Talk to dieters and you'll find they're often a pretty cynical lot. They've been burned before, and they readily acknowledge that they'll probably be burned again. To some, a new diet is just another roll of the dice. This is deplorable, not only because it's dangerous to play dice with one's health but also because it doesn't take much effort to replace resignation and cynicism with a little productive investigative work.

Asking the right questions and pondering the answers at the outset will help you to (a) avoid wasting time, money, and energy on bad diets and (b) make better use of good diets, should you stumble on any. You can't make optimal use of anything unless you understand how it works — or is supposed to work.

In this chapter, then, I provide you with some of the information that I believe makes the Feel Full Diet worth your time. I'm not going to claim that this diet is the very model of scientific purity. The truth is that it's extremely difficult to test a diet rigorously. To do so would take five or ten years, cost millions of dollars, and involve hundreds of "experimental" and "control" volunteers. Only very recently has the government begun to fund such ambitious studies, and then not for weight loss but for disease prevention.

The Feel Full Diet, nonetheless, is on a firmer foundation than most, possibly all, weight-loss diets. It is distinguished from most of the fad diets by the following:

1. The theory upon which the diet is based is supported by a large body of scientific and medical literature from a wide range of independent sources.

2. My own research on matters contributing to the diet has been widely published in scientific and medical journals that adhere to close professional scrutiny before accepting anything for publication.

3. My specialized training as an M.D. is in gastroenterol-

ogy, which focuses on human metabolism, nutrition, digestion, diet, and the like.

4. Many of the assumptions of this diet have been confirmed by careful animal and human experimentation.

5. The diet has been tried, in a clinical hospital setting, on a large number of people, and used by many others with excellent results. It may come as a surprise to many of you to learn that some very well-known fad diets were tried on *no one* before being taken to "market."

Let's look now at some of the findings that helped me develop the Feel Full Diet.

OBESITY—A HORMONE PROBLEM AFTER ALL?

Remember when overweight folks used to wonder if their obesity had some "glandular" or hormonal basis? Most doctors—and most lean people—scoffed at this notion. They dismissed it as just another feeble excuse for overeating by people they believed to be seriously lacking in willpower. The obese person brave enough to suggest "hormones" to his or her doctor was (and often still is) told: "Less than 1 percent of all cases of obesity are caused by hormonal disturbances, so you can forget that. Your problem is simple: you eat too much. Hormones have nothing to do with it."

What these doctors were referring to is just one hormone— the thyroid hormone. Well, the problem certainly *is* eating too much. But is it true that hormones have *nothing* to do with it in most cases? The best evidence now indicates that hormones have a *lot* to do with how we eat—and not just in rare cases. One or more biochemical, hormone-related defects may well be present in *many* obese people, defects that block the feeling of fullness or slow body metabolism and thus encourage overeating.

In the last chapter, I discussed the hormone CCK, which I

have labeled a "satiety" hormone—one that signals fullness in normal-weight people. Is there really any evidence that CCK is a "feel full" hormone? Yes, lots of it.

I was the first person to discover a CCK "antagonist," that is, a substance that *blocks* the effects of CCK on all of the organs it normally affects, including the brain, pancreas, and gallbladder. Finding a CCK blocker has made it much easier to study and confirm the effects that internally produced CCK has on these various organs. It has made it easier to show that CCK really is a satiety hormone.

Among other experiments, my coworkers and I have injected this CCK blocker into the brains of sheep, stopping the hormone's effects right in the "control center." With CCK—the hormone that we postulated could turn off hunger—thus neutralized, the sheep did exactly what we predicted they would do: they overate significantly.

Later we used yet another CCK blocker, one that didn't have to be injected but could be given orally. When we fed this CCK inhibitor to rats, they also overate. Such experiments make it very evident that the body's own CCK is important in regulating the rate of food intake in every animal tested, including man. CCK is truly a "feel full" hormone.

But CCK is not the only hormone that has been found to stimulate the feeling of fullness. Glucagon, a hormone that causes the blood sugar to increase, has also been shown to decrease food intake in experimental animals. Other examples are bombesin, or gastrin-releasing peptide, and somatostatin, although not nearly as much information is available on these hormones, and their effect on food intake in humans is not yet known.

DOES A CCK IMBALANCE CAUSE OBESITY?

The research findings related above don't directly prove that CCK defects—such as an insufficient amount of the hormone

—*cause* obesity. A CCK abnormality, however, could be involved in obesity in a major way. To find out to what extent—and more precisely *how*—CCK disturbances contribute to overeating, we conducted still other experiments, some of which yielded exciting results.

My associates and I studied both lean rats and overweight rats. You might expect that the overweight rats would produce less CCK than the lean rats and that this might be the key to the problem. But that wasn't the case. We found that both fat and skinny rats produced normal amounts of CCK. Yet we did find that in the overweight rats all of the functions of CCK were markedly diminished. In other words, though present in normal amounts in the obese rats, the CCK just didn't seem to be doing its job. It didn't seem to be getting to its target organs in sufficient amounts to make them work properly. The pancreases of these animals, for example, didn't react to CCK as responsively as they should have.

We found that even when we injected extra CCK into the overweight rats they still didn't decrease their food intake as much as their lean littermates did when they were given extra CCK. This held true even though we injected the obese animals with more CCK than we did the lean rats.

Why doesn't CCK work as well in overweight animals? Here we made perhaps our most startling discovery. By "tagging" (coupling) CCK with a special radioactive material we were able to trace in greater detail its progress and action in the body. We discovered by this process that the obese animals we studied have only one-fourth the normal number of CCK "receptors." These receptors are protein structures on the surface of cells in various parts of the digestive tract. They serve as points of attachment by which the CCK binds to cells in the pancreas, stomach, and other target organs.

What we found then was that even though CCK levels are normal in obese animals, the hormone can't work as effectively as it does in lean animals because there aren't enough receptors to enable adequate quantities of the chemical to exert its effects.

It is this lack of CCK receptors that constitutes the hormone-related biochemical defect that may be at the base of overeating in obese rats.

The situation here is rather like that seen in adult-onset diabetes. As you know, most of these diabetics have to take extra insulin on a regular basis to keep their metabolism or glucose level on an even keel. This is true even though they produce normal amounts of insulin. What they lack is an adequate number of insulin receptors. And so to maintain a normal blood sugar they require more than normal amounts of insulin to find and bind to the limited number of receptors.

The same holds true with respect to CCK and the obese animals we studied. We did finally succeed in getting them to stop eating so much (followed by significant weight loss), but to do this we had to increase the supply of CCK in their systems substantially. Studies at Mt. Sinai Hospital in New York and more recently in my laboratory indicate that obese humans as well as obese laboratory animals do not respond normally to CCK. These data provide good support for our hypothesis that obesity in humans may be related to one or more biochemical defects.

CAN THE BIOCHEMICAL DEFECT BE CORRECTED?

We have already shown that by introducing CCK *blockers* into the system, we can get animals to overeat. And by *injecting* CCK into them we can, eventually, get them to *stop* overeating. Is there anything else—more practical—that we can do?

I hear from a lot of overweight people who tell me they would gladly take CCK pills or injections on a daily basis for the rest of their lives if it would help them stop eating. Various CCK pills have, in fact, been marketed through health-food stores and the like. Unfortunately, these pills are worthless. CCK taken *by mouth* is degraded (broken down) in the digestive system before it can have any useful effect in the body. *Injected* CCK can be effective for a while, but studies on long-term safety and effectiveness have not yet been performed.

We *have* now discovered some other means of manipulating CCK, the most important of which are dietary and are, of course, the subject of this book. In addition to diet, however, we are looking at substances that might eventually (perhaps ten years from now) become the basis for a genuinely effective antiobesity drug. We've already shown, in experiments, that substances that inhibit the action of an enzyme called trypsin can diminish food intake. This is so because trypsin is itself a CCK blocker. It's an enzyme that occurs naturally in the body and is the body's mechanism for "switching off" CCK after its work is done. When the action of this enzyme was inhibited we found that the body would keep on producing CCK and thus inhibit hunger in obese animals.

But after having looked at everything likely to have any effect on CCK, I have concluded that *the only safe and effective long-term method for favorably manipulating the hormone in humans at the present time is dietary.*

The experimental data related to CCK and humans are not as well developed as for other animals. The reason is simple enough: it's easier, safer, and less expensive to do experiments on lower animals. Nonetheless, experiments have been conducted in which CCK has been injected into both lean and obese humans. Such injections resulted in markedly decreased food intake. In addition, we have shown that gallbladders from obese humans don't contract as well in response to CCK as those from lean humans. This doesn't prove but suggests that obese humans are very much like the obese rats we studied in this respect.

Others have shown that obese humans secrete smaller quantities of pancreatic enzymes in response to CCK—again similar to what we have shown in rats. Interestingly, when overweight humans in some of this work lost many of their excess pounds, their pancreatic functions returned to normal. This suggests that the biochemical defect may be *reversible* to some degree—that as significant weight loss occurs the body may become more responsive to CCK. This in turn could make it possible for the once overweight person to feel full after eating smaller meals.

In any event, from all this work it became evident to me that a diet designed to increase the *body's own* supply of CCK at strategic intervals related to food intake was the way to go. The research left no doubt about CCK's ability to stimulate a feeling of fullness and therefore turn off hunger. But it was also clear that just adding CCK to the diet wouldn't work at all. And injecting it may be neither safe nor effective in the long run.

Diet appeared to be the only way to get the body to do what we wanted it to do—in a natural and safe way. In the next two chapters you'll meet some of the people who have used this diet, and you can judge for yourself how effective this diet has been —ridding people both of excess pounds and of unnecessary and unwarranted guilt. Later chapters will describe the diet itself in detail, and you'll learn how and why this diet can enable you to manipulate the "feel full" mechanisms you've learned about in this chapter.

3

Case Histories—
Losing the Pounds

LOSING WEIGHT WITH *LESS* WILLPOWER

"ALL IT TAKES to lose weight is willpower." How many times have you heard that? How many times have you believed it? Probably more than you care to remember. I'll dispell some of the myths that promote the idea that most obesity has a psychological basis in the next chapter. Right now let's focus on losing weight—not with willpower but by *feeling full*. If you've read the preceding chapters you know that the lack of sensation of fullness is one of the most important reasons people fail to curb calorie intake.

One woman with a long-standing weight problem summed it all up very neatly: "To lose weight you've got to cut the calories. There's no way around that. And I did cut calories on at least a dozen different diets—and I also gained it all back. The reason wasn't a lack of willpower. It was that I *never* felt satisfied. I *never* felt full."

Most diets fail to consider the satiety aspect and will severely restrict fat intake, making potato chips, ice cream, and pepperoni "forbidden food." The Feel Full Diet understands the need for a certain amount of fat in the diet to make one feel satisfied. That's part of the reason people don't feel deprived on this diet.

What follows are summaries of the experiences of several satisfied individuals, people who were once overweight but who finally achieved that elusive full feeling using our diet. All these individuals have not only lost significant amounts of weight but also give every indication that they will be able to keep the pounds off permanently. These people are typical of those using the Feel Full Diet. Names and backgrounds have been changed to protect identities.

"FULL? I DIDN'T KNOW THE MEANING OF THE WORD."

Clare was overweight "for as long as I can remember." So were her mother and sisters. She began dieting in her teens, but nothing worked for very long. For years she suffered misplaced guilt and shame, which I'll discuss in the next chapter. At one point she even concluded that being fat was a family curse.

"The whole idea of being hungry all the time was something I lived with day in and day out—and well into the night, too. As for being full, I didn't know the meaning of the word."

Clare was in her forties, 5 feet 7 inches tall, and weighed about 175 pounds, when she started on the Feel Full Diet. She'd heard about it through an acquaintance of mine and decided to try it on her own.

"It appealed to me," she recalls, "because it seemed to have some scientific basis, not just somebody out in Hollywood telling me that if I eat kiwi all day I'll end up looking like Joan Collins. Besides, I'd long since promised that if I could look one-fourth as svelte as Joan Collins I'd stand naked in the middle of Times Square and sing the 'Hallelujah Chorus.' My husband, God bless him, said he'd pay for the orchestra."

The diet appealed for other reasons, too. "I really liked this idea of the satietizer. It seemed a little strange at first—the idea that eating a higher-fat snack before lunch or dinner would actually make me want to eat less when it came to the main course. But it also made sense when I learned about CCK and some of the other hormones that control so many of our eating habits. I understood that getting that fat or protein content into the system at just the right time was the key. And, hey, I wasn't about to complain if somebody said I could lose weight eating shrimp in sour cream, peanut butter-honey balls, miniature pizzas, deviled eggs, nachos with cheese, and a whole lot of other really fantastic stuff."

Clare began making large batches of some of her favorite satietizers. She freezes some of them and often takes them to work with her. As lunch approaches she eats one at her desk, timing it so that she doesn't get to the restaurant for her main course until half an hour later. (I'll say more about eating out in the Feel Full Diet later.)

Clare says the fact that she was able to keep on eating, although in reduced quantities, so many of foods she had always loved made the Feel Full Diet easy for her to adapt to right from the beginning. "Try one of those diets where you have to eat nothing but grapefruit or sardines all day and you'll discover real fast how hard dieting can be. This diet wasn't like that. And if I ate the satietizers when I was supposed to, waited the twenty to thirty minutes, and then sat down again for the main course, I found I *could* resist eating too much. I genuinely did begin to experience what I'd previously thought was a myth—fullness. There was a hint of it at first. And it got stronger each day I stayed on the diet. As I began to lose the pounds, I felt it more and more. And, meanwhile, though I wasn't gorging on foods I'd always loved, I was still getting a taste of them every day."

The main courses were no chore, either, Clare observes. "I was aware of the need to reduce fat intake in my diet overall, and this approach—higher-fat satietizer, lower-fat main meal —certainly made it easier for me. Now I follow most of the guidelines you've developed with respect to the six food groups [more details in later chapters] and have no difficulty constructing meals both I and my husband and even our kids find tasty and interesting. Believe me, my family finds this diet a real relief compared with most of the ones I've been on. What I used to hear was, 'Oh, no, Mom's on a new diet; let's go to Burger King.' Now, more often, it's 'What's for dinner, Mom?'"

Clare averaged 800 to 1000 calories per day on the Feel Full Diet. She stayed at that level for nearly seven months and in that time span lost more than 50 pounds—about 2 pounds per week. She suffered a couple of very short-term "lapses" during holiday periods but otherwise found it "smooth sailing." She is now on a maintenance program that permits her to consume 1500 calories per day and is holding her weight close to 125 pounds. She has had no difficulty, she reports, holding at that weight for several months now.

"One of the best things about this diet," Clare adds, "apart from the fact that it actually works, is that I never felt irritable on it. And there was no fatigue, either, except in the very beginning, when there was a little at the 800-calorie level. That went away fast."

But best of all, she concludes, is "the fact that I can now say 'I'm full' at the end of a meal and really mean it for the first time in my life."

Okay. So what about that promise to stand naked in the middle of Times Square and sing the "Hallelujah Chorus"?

"Ah, but you didn't listen carefully," Clare responds. "That promise was good only if I ended up looking *one-fourth* as svelte as Joan Collins. I'd say I did better than that, wouldn't you? So, I'm off the hook."

Too bad for Times Square.

"I ALREADY HAD THREE SIZES OF SHIRTS."

Bob, a busy executive in his late forties, was abruptly told by his doctor that it was time to lose weight. Actually, it was past time. Bob acknowledges that he'd been a bit overweight for some time and had started to gain even faster after he quit smoking a few years ago. Over the last decade he'd made some "halfhearted attempts" to shed some pounds, but nothing came of these efforts. Instead, he kept gaining weight.

It wasn't just the doctor who prodded Bob into trying the Feel Full Diet. "Every time I looked in my closet," he says, "I realized I was either going to have to lose some weight or buy some more shirts. And I already had three different sizes hanging in there!"

Bob took quickly to the idea of the satietizer. There was one he liked so much and that seemed to work so well for him that he used it nearly every day. This was the peanut butter and celery satietizer. Like Clare, Bob liked the underlying scientific rationale for the Feel Full Diet. He also liked the fact that "the diet is nutritionally well-balanced." Bob had long since concluded that crash diets—on which you lose large amounts of weight in short periods of time—are dangerous and ineffective in the long run. The idea of slower but surer (in the sense of being more permanent) weight loss appealed to Bob.

Bob started out on a 1300- to 1400-calorie diet, fairly typical for dieting males. (Later chapters will explain the different calorie-level options suitable for men and women.) After the third week, however, he cut back to 1200 calories because, as he puts it, "I discovered I really liked the idea of losing weight. I was losing it without hunger so I decided to cut back a little further." He did this and still did not experience any difficulty with hunger. In addition, he started exercising moderately. He'd been losing one to two pounds per week on the diet and, not surprisingly, began losing even more after he started exercising. (Exercise is optional for most dieters, but I highly recommend it in combination with dieting for reasons I'll explain in a subsequent chapter on exercise. For some people exercise is vital.)

In a few months, Bob, who is 5 feet 6 inches tall, dropped from over 160 pounds to 130 pounds. He experienced no fatigue during the weight-loss period. "In fact, I felt great," he says. "I really enjoyed having people come up to me and say, 'Have you been on a diet? You look wonderful.' And though I've been happily married for twenty-six years, I certainly didn't mind when attractive young women suddenly began telling me, 'You really look good.'"

Another bonus: "I'm wearing shirts I haven't been able to wear in years."

"The diet has really worked for me," Bob says. "I don't get hungry on this diet. And overall the diet has led me to change my attitude about eating. I like being the weight I am now, and I believe I will stick with many of these changes in eating style for the rest of my life. It isn't just the satietizer. It's also the changes in the main courses, in everything I eat and how I eat. In many ways I don't think of this as a diet but as a change in behavior."

Bob has found, like many others, that as he has lost weight and gone on to a maintenance diet he can now control his food intake *without* always having a satietizer before a main meal. Increasingly, Bob finds he can do without the satietizer, suggesting that perhaps there has been a reversal or at least a partial reversal in the biochemical defect that previously prevented him from feeling full at the appropriate time. You'll recall from the preceding chapters that the experimental data hint that such a reversal may be possible.

Some other features of the Feel Full Diet Bob particularly likes are the six food groups rather than four and the fact that amounts of food are expressed in "servings" rather than strictly in calories. Many people comment favorably on these facets of the diet. They say it makes it easier to get balanced fare that is lower in fat and higher in healthy fiber and complex carbohydrates (which are *not* fattening, as you'll see). Converting calories to typical serving sizes makes it easier for many to monitor their daily food intake. You'll get more details on this in the chapter dealing with main courses.

Because the diet worked so well for Bob, his wife decided to try it, too. She has a somewhat more severe weight problem and some medical difficulties that complicate dieting. Nonetheless, she is also steadily losing weight.

"It's great," Bob concludes, "finally being able to say, 'Sorry, I can't finish the macaroni and cheese.'"

"MY HUSBAND NEVER THOUGHT I WOULD DO IT."

Rose had been putting on weight for the last ten years. In her mid-fifties she found herself nearly 20 pounds heavier than she wanted to be, but after a decade of fighting excess pounds, going from about 140 to 120 "seemed unrealistic." Nonetheless, that was the goal she set for herself when she started the Feel Full Diet. She'd set such goals before. She had tried many other diets, including several of the trendy "crash" diets.

"I liked this diet much better right from the start," she states. "This one is much easier. The satietizers have a definite effect. In fact, I often carry them with me in little baggies. The whole diet made sense to me. I felt better on it right from the start. There were no bad side effects, only good ones." A few months after starting her diet, Rose was very near her "unrealistic" goal of 120 pounds and should arrive there any day now.

Like Bob, Rose feels that this diet "changes your behavior or lifestyle, so that you eat in a different way that will stick with you for a very long time, probably permanently." Rose particularly likes the fact that she can still eat many of the foods that other diets would have denied her. "I love chocolate," she says. "And by following the guidelines, I can still work a little chocolate into my diet without really cheating. That's one of the great things about this program. It's not as rigid as many of the others. You get a good variety of foods. It's not monotonous, and it doesn't make you feel guilty about eating things you like."

Rose feels that the satietizers have been particularly effective in subduing her enthusiasm for sweets and snacks. "I used to be the kind of person who when I'd go into a restaurant would look at the dessert menu *first* and worry about the main course later. Or when I'd come home in the afternoon at 3:00 I'd start grabbing candy and crackers and keep it up until dinner at 5:30. Now I find that a satietizer in the late afternoon will hold me until dinner, and I no longer feel the urge for all the snacks. That's really been remarkable. And, in fact, that's exactly why my husband never thought I would do it, why he thought I'd never lose the weight—because I was always such a nosher. He knew how many other diets I'd gone on and how the snacks had always won out. Not this time."

"IT ALL SEEMED SO EASY."

Sheldon was in his sixties when his surgeon told him he'd better lose some weight. He was 5 feet 10 inches tall and weighed 232 pounds. "I'd been overweight for twenty years," he observes. "I started gaining weight the day I married."

In less than two and a half months on the Feel Full Diet, Sheldon lost 40 pounds. "During this entire period," he says, "I couldn't believe I was losing weight." It all seemed so easy and, he recalls, so long as he did not go below 1300 calories a day he experienced no fatigue or grouchiness.

He reports that the satietizers were very tasty, not a bother, and that he used them "95 percent of the time." He and his wife often dine out. "Sometimes I take a satietizer along and eat it in the car if we're going out to dinner."

Like Rose, Sheldon reports that the satietizers have been effective not only in helping him eat less during the main course but also have made it easier for him to resist snacking. He is particularly fond of those satietizers that include peanut butter or shrimp. (You'll be relieved to learn, however, that so far we haven't combined those two items!)

Like most of the others on the Feel Full Diet, Sheldon is happy with the mixed variety of foods the regimen provides. His way of eating has changed "quite a lot," he says, but he is happy that he can still sample many old favorites. His wife, inspired by his success, has now also gone on the diet and, at last report, had shed twenty-five pounds.

"Both of us," Sheldon notes, "still like some dessert now and then. When we eat out we sometimes order one portion, and both of us take a bite and then let it go. We have that one taste and then we don't feel like we're being cheated."

Sheldon concludes: "I can live very well with this diet. I see it as a long-term commitment." And one, as he pointed out in the beginning, that hasn't been at all difficult to make—and keep.

"DON'T EAT THAT! YOU'LL SPOIL YOUR APPETITE!"

The case histories related above are typical of those who use the Feel Full Diet. Obviously the diet does not work exactly the same for every individual. We've had some failures, too. Most of my patients enjoy the satietizers and do not find it inconvenient to wait twenty or thirty minutes before starting the main course. Occasionally, though, I'll find some individuals who can't adapt to this schedule, and their dieting efforts are less successful. If you *do* adhere to the proper schedule and restrict calories as directed later in this book, you *will* lose weight— and with less hunger than you've experienced on other diets. The success stories I've related here convince me of that, especially when coupled with the scientific data outlined in the preceding chapters.

Actually, if you think about it, you can probably come up

with some of your own case histories in support of this diet. Almost all of us can remember our mothers repeatedly scolding, "Don't eat that! You'll spoil your appetite." This admonition was usually in response to spotting us munching on carbohydrates, mainly potato chips, cheese, or other "rich" (that is, high-fat) foods shortly before lunch or dinner. And unless you're one of those people who can't *ever* recall what it was like to feel full, you know your mother was often right. By the time dinner rolled around, your appetite *had* sagged. Had you eaten a carrot, however, instead of a cookie, your mother would probably have fainted or at least said nothing and you would still have been hungry when the main course arrived. Some of you may remember going to an expensive restaurant, ordering an "appetizer," and being unable to finish the entrée that was served twenty minutes later.

It isn't, as I've noted, just the act of snacking before a main course that curbs appetite. It's *what* you eat, *how much* you eat, and *when*.

But before we get into the specifics of the diet itself, let's grab a little more inspiration. In the next chapter we'll talk not only about how people like you have lost weight but also how they've lost their guilt and stopped punishing themselves in the process for something that really isn't their fault.

4

Stop Punishing Yourself: Losing the Guilt

"FOR TOO MANY YEARS I'VE BEEN HATING MYSELF..."

YOU'D HAVE TO read the mail I get from people who are overweight to begin fully to grasp the intense anguish, guilt, and self-hatred that afflicts so many who are obese. Every time an article or news item appears about my work showing that obesity has a biochemical rather than a psychological basis, mail floods in. Most express deep relief that the facts about obesity are finally coming to light.

"It's terrible enough," one woman wrote, "that we must carry this extra weight, which so repulses both society and ourselves, but that we should also have to bear this burden of guilt and shame for something that is not really our fault is intolerable."

A group of women combined forces to write me: "At last

27

someone knows the true reason for obesity. Please let us volunteer for your research on the chemical defect and overweight. We have suffered so long and so much.... Please help us."

Another woman wrote to describe her decades-long, truly Herculean efforts to lose weight. These failed efforts had been greeted, by those who had never known what it is to feel incessant hunger, with scorn and derision. Yet this woman still exhibited a fighting spirit and, buoyed by what she had read of our research, concluded: "Being heavy *has* to be a chemical imbalance, the same as having any other medical problem. Keep up the good and great work."

Yet another woman wrote of her extreme depression over her failure to lose weight: "I have been on more diets than there are pages in a phone book. I always lose, but in a short time I gain back the weight and then some...for too many years I have been hating myself."

A woman who described her appetite as "unbelievable" recounted the anguish she has experienced because of her obesity. Much of this has been caused by the reaction of others. Despite her concerted efforts to lose weight over the years, she writes, "My husband makes fun of me, and my mother is very critical." Like many others who have written to me, this woman feels that there is always the smug suggestion in the air, when the lean survey the fat, that obese people secretly *like* being the way they are—otherwise they'd just lose weight. But as this woman put it, simply but eloquently, in all capital letters: "I DO NOT WANT TO BE FAT!"

Listen up, society. This woman is right. I've never met a single overweight person who really liked being that way, though a *few*, to put up a happy front, will claim they do. There is no myth more false than that of a "jolly" fat man or woman. You know as well as I that they are laughing on the outside and crying on the inside.

A woman wrote me that both she and her daughter are extremely overweight. "It's very upsetting," she said, "because I know my daughter will suffer like I have." She went on to describe her efforts at losing weight. Hunger, she said, was always with her. "I am always searching for something. It's as if there is always something missing—never feeling full, never feeling satisfied. *It's enough to drive a sane person crazy.* I have been to doctors time and time again with no help. All tests say everything is fine. I am not lacking, they say, in anything except willpower."

There's that word—*willpower*. Almost all my patients say that they have repeatedly been accused of lacking willpower. This is not only a bum rap, it's a cruel and hypocritical one about which I'll have more to say shortly.

THE WHY-AM-I-OVERWEIGHT QUIZ

Having survived college, medical school, and certifying boards in internal medicine and gastroenterology, I automatically find myself asking questions in the multiple-choice format. My students at Jefferson Medical College will attest to that. Now, here's a multiple-choice quiz for *you*:

I became fat for the following reason(s):
   A. I have no self-control or willpower
   B. I just love eating
   C. I have a psychological disorder
   D. All of the above
   E. None of the above

Most people taking this quiz, provided they hadn't read this book, would answer D, "All of the above," or at least one of the other choices (A, B, or C) if they thought they were being "honest" or "objective" about themselves. It's no secret to me that the overweight are among the first to believe the lies about themselves that society as a whole promotes. After all, they've heard these myths all their lives. They are constantly being reminded, first by others and then by themselves, that their girth is self-inflicted.

"How can you do that to yourself?" "Don't you have any self-respect?" "If you don't want to be fat, why don't you just stop eating?" You have heard this and felt this all your overweight life, and you still don't have the answer.

What *is* the right answer? A, B, C, D, or E? The answer in virtually 100 percent of all cases of the common form of obesity, is E—*none of the above!* Sadly, even after some learn that this is the case, they still do not entirely believe it. They want to believe, but they are so down on themselves, after all those years of negative conditioning, that they have trouble letting go of the myths.

It's vital that you *do* let go of these myths, however, because as long as you cling to them, *no* diet program can work effectively for you. It's important that the people close to you *also* understand the real causes of obesity so that they can set aside their prejudices and give you the support you so badly need. Thus I strongly suggest that you and your family and friends read this chapter.

The best way to dispel the myths is to take them apart. Let's analyze each potential answer in the quiz separately.

"A.   I HAVE NO SELF-CONTROL OR WILLPOWER"

To understand the willpower issue, we have to go back to Chapter 1, "What Makes You Hungry? What Makes You Full?" In reality, both thin and fat people behave the same way when it comes to eating. They start eating when they get hungry, and they stop eating when they feel full. But we now know that many overweight people don't sense "fullness" as clearly as lean people do. That's why, as explained in Chapter 2, overeating can occur in some people before the fullness signals register in the brain.

The important thing to remember here is that lean people eat less than you do *only* because they sense fullness earlier and more clearly. It has nothing to do with "superior" willpower. Their willpower, in fact, is never tested. That's why I say they are being hypocritical when they criticize the overweight in this context.

Willpower—or rather the lack of it—is definitely *not a cause* of obesity. It can be argued that it is a factor in the *treatment* of obesity. It is true that highly motivated fat people lose more weight than those with less motivation. But, again, this is a treatment issue and must not be confused with the cause of obesity. The purpose of the Feel Full Diet is to cut down on the need for willpower by making low-calorie meals more satisfying.

Lack of willpower does *not* explain how you developed your weight problem.

"B.   I JUST LOVE EATING"

Let me tell all of you heavy folks reading this book a closely guarded secret: thin people love to eat, too! In fact, for many of us, it's a favorite pastime. Eating is so enjoyable we take any and every opportunity to arrange our lives and schedules around food. We constantly conspire to consummate business deals over consommé and launch love affairs over lunch.

It may surprise you to learn, too, that many thin people actually eat as much as if not more than you do. Whether the individual becomes thin or fat in these instances depends upon his or her body metabolism. Thin: lucky. Fat: unlucky. Again, not your fault.

Thin people who eat a lot are said to have "hearty" appetites. While the skinnies bolt down the food in ravenous gulps, their mothers gleefully chorus: "God love 'em!" But when the heavies gather enough courage to creep "out of the closet" long enough to down a big meal in front of family and friends, they are greeted with a chorus of derision or at least a flock of raised eyebrows on lean foreheads. What is considered hearty in one is described as gluttony in another. But, in reality, it's exactly the same thing.

So, I'm sorry, just because you love to eat doesn't make you different from anyone else. It *doesn't* explain how you became overweight.

"C. I HAVE A PSYCHOLOGICAL DISORDER"

Psychological problems were, until very recently, believed to be the primary causes of obesity. Both physicians and lay people believed this, and many still do. People were thought to be overweight because they were "sublimating" various emotions, because they were sexually "starved" or otherwise disturbed, because they had received faulty toilet training, because they were shy and couldn't interact with other people constructively, because they were violent, because they'd experienced some terrible trauma or were neglected in childhood, because they were self-destructive, because they'd learned "bad eating habits" early in life, because they'd never learned to cope with stress, and so on. There were—and, alas, are—as many theories as there are different schools of psychology.

And because the idea that psychological problems cause obesity took root so early, psychologists and psychiatrists are the ones who have, typically, been given the responsibility of treating the overweight. Most of the research papers related to obesity have been written over the years by psychiatrists and psychologists. They have dominated the field, and it has only been in recent times that basic scientists and physicians from other fields (physiology, biochemistry, endocrinology, gastroenterology) have shed new light on the problem.

And, frankly, until recently, many of us in those other fields were content to leave this vexing problem to the psychiatrists. We were so ignorant, for so long, of the real causes of obesity that it was very convenient to pass the buck to the psychology sector. This is not unusual in medicine. In many instances when we haven't been able to find a physical cause for a disease or disorder, we simply conclude that it's "all in the head" and therefore psychological in origin. Sometimes we later do discover a physical cause, and then there's a lot of embarrassment and sometimes denial.

In addition, however, the issue of the source of obesity was badly clouded because the overweight often *do* develop psychological problems. These problems, however, may not be the cause but the *result* of obesity. This important distinction was finally officially recognized by experts participating in a National Institutes of Health (NIH) consensus-development conference on obesity in 1985. Dr. Albert J. Stunkard, a leading authority on obesity from the University of Pennsylvania, told the conference that these psychological problems develop as a consequence of obesity but are not a cause of it. They result, he added, because of society's negative attitudes toward being overweight and also "through the effects of dieting." Dr. Stunkard, by the way, is a psychiatrist, showing that attitudes are changing in his field as well.

Dr. Stunkard illustrated the pervasive negative prejudice against the obese by citing studies in which children and adults were shown silhouettes of obese children, lean children, and obviously handicapped children. A group of six-year-olds described the fat children as "ugly," "stupid," "cheater," "liar," and "dirty." And both children and adults said they would befriend the lean or handicapped children they viewed in silhouettes before they would the fat children.

This deep-seated prejudice against excess pounds, Dr. Stunkard reported, is "not only uniform among blacks and whites and persons from urban and rural settings but it is observed among the obese themselves."

Little wonder that psychological problems develop! But, remember, these are the result and not the cause of obesity. You are not fat because you are bad or somehow disturbed mentally. It is vital that you recognize this. Otherwise even the *best* diet is going to be an uphill battle. It's very difficult to succeed at anything if you don't feel good about yourself.

You should also be aware, as Dr. Stunkard suggested, that *dieting itself* can make you feel bad, not just physically bad but mentally bad. This isn't surprising given the way many fad diets are constructed. If you go on a crash diet that doesn't provide enough calories even to keep basic metabolic functions operating properly, of course you're going to get into trouble. That's why so many diets leave people feeling disoriented, lightheaded, irritable, and fatigued. This happens, too, when the diet does not deliver a proper *balance* of macronutrients (fat, protein, carbohydrates) and micronutrients (vitamins, minerals, amino acids). Diets that leave people feeling hungry or somehow lacking in something are just naturally going to produce unhappy people.

The key here is to recognize that the unhappiness is attributable to the diet and not to some personality disorder within yourself. And the solution, as this book keeps suggesting, is to find a diet that makes you feel full! As the case histories in the preceding chapter demonstrated, dieters do not become angry, irritated, or fatigued while using the Feel Full Diet. This is because it provides ample calories, mixed nutrients, and, most important, that full feeling.

One issue remains to be dealt with under the general heading of psychology. This is stress. Many people claim that stress is responsible for overeating and cite this as evidence that obesity does, in fact, have a psychological basis. It is certainly true that some people do eat more when they are having emotional difficulties, trouble at work, marriage or relationship problems, and the like. Remember, though, that this is as true of lean people as it is of the overweight. And many of those stressed-out, overeating, lean individuals never do become obese. There is something far more fundamental than stress at work here, and numerous experiments have shown that that "something" is biochemical in nature. Even overeating that is experimentally induced through the presence of constant stress can be halted by introducing adequate amounts of the fullness hormone CCK.

Yes, it is easier to diet when stress is reduced or eliminated. Make every effort to reduce stressful situations in your life. One of the best ways to start is to shed any guilt you might have about being overweight. That, more than anything else, will set the stage for a successful weight-reduction program.

WHERE DID THE REAL CAUSE OF OBESITY ORIGINATE?

Now that you know what doesn't cause obesity you are probably wondering where the real cause—these biochemical defects—came from. How is it that 34 million people in the United States have these defects? The answers aren't definitely known yet, but genetics, shaped in part by environment, appear to be responsible. We've all noticed that heavy parents tend to have heavy offspring—not always, to be sure, but often enough to make it evident that there's such a thing as a "heavy" gene. In addition, heavy individuals often have heavy spouses, further compounding the genetic factor.

The type of inheritance observed in obesity is called "multifactorial." In simple terms this means that genes which code for obesity can be transmitted from parent to child but in unpredictable ways. No one knows the exact risk a child has of becoming obese, but the risk is clearly higher than normal if one or both parents is overweight. Further evidence for a genetic rather than an environmental cause of human obesity comes from a recent study at the University of Pennsylvania. Dr. Stunkard and his coworkers found that the weight of adopted children correlate much better with the body type of their biologic parents (especially the mother) than their adoptive parents. Many people overlook this genetic component and instead accuse obese parents of stuffing their children the same way they supposedly stuff themselves.

The concept of evolutionary "natural selection," involving

circumstances that enable some individuals to survive and perpetuate themselves better than others, may also help explain why so many are overweight today. Much of human history has been characterized by periods of severe famine. Those individuals who had the ability to eat more than normal during times of plenty and to store the excess in the form of fat were more likely to survive, it has been argued, during times when food was in short supply. This natural selection may have promoted what some have called the "thrifty" gene (so called because it causes highly efficient use of nutrients by the body), one that actually encourages obesity.

Well, the thrifty gene may have come in handy during the Ice Age or any number of famines, but in America today it results in nothing but unwanted excess baggage.

Fortunately, the biochemical bases of obesity are slowly being exposed. As scientists from diverse disciplines recognize that obesity is *not* the result of excessive love of food, lack of willpower, or psychological disturbances, and as even an official government body (the NIH consensus conference) has officially declared that obesity is a *physical disease,* we can raise our expectations for finding effective solutions to this very serious problem. Obesity contributes to hundreds of thousands of premature deaths annually. It is a significant factor in cardiovascular disease (which can lead to heart attacks and strokes), hypertension (high blood pressure), adult-onset diabetes, cancer of the breast, cancer of the uterus, cancer of the prostate, cancers of the colon and rectum, and, as we've seen, it can also result in serious psychological problems.

When Dr. Jules Hirsch, chairman of the NIH conference on obesity, said that obesity is a disease and "not a condition like loneliness," that signaled a real social and scientific breakthrough—and a triumph for all of you who are struggling with both pounds and prejudice.

Now, in a positive, guilt-free frame of mind, let's learn a simple but effective new way of eating that takes advantage of some of this important new knowledge. On to the Feel Full Diet itself. Actually, without knowing it, you've already begun, for this is a diet that begins—and ends—in the mind, the full cooperation of which is vital for permanent weight loss and maintenance.

5

The Diet Itself:
Summary and Goals

HIGHLIGHTS OF THE FEEL FULL DIET

HERE, IN BRIEF, are some of the most important features of
the Feel Full Diet:

• Calories *are* restricted. Diet authors who tell you calories
don't count are peddling hot air. There's no way around it: you
can't cut pounds without cutting calories.

• Caloric allotments, however, are generous on the Feel Full
Diet—approximately 1200 calories per day for women and
about 1300 calories per day for men on the standard program. For women who want faster results there is an optional
1000-calories-per-day program. For men who find the standard
male 1300 calories program too restrictive, there is an optional
1800-calories-per-day alternative.

• Satietizers precede lunch and dinner. The satietizers, ac-
counting for about 300 calories per day for women and 400

calories per day for men, are relatively high in fat and protein and are designed to stimulate the "feel full" hormones.

• Main courses, however, are lower in fat than typical American fare. *Overall* the Feel Full Diet encourages a reduction in the consumption of fat, and particularly the saturated fats and cholesterol that have been implicated in so many diseases. Concurrently, the Feel Full Diet encourages an increase in the consumption of complex carbohydrates and foods rich in fiber. The Feel Full Diet, however, is highly *flexible*. As long as you stay within caloric guidelines and follow the timing procedure related to satietizers and main courses, you can pick and choose from a variety of foods.

• *Timing* of food consumption is a crucial factor in the Feel Full Diet. To activate the "feel full" hormones properly you must follow the prescribed procedures—really quite simple— with respect to satietizer, *intrameal* interval, and *main course,* all to be described in more detail in subsequent chapters.

• Exercise is an optional part of the Feel Full Diet program but one that will have lasting benefits for almost everybody and may be necessary for certain individuals who will be identified. Exercise helps you favorably regulate your metabolic set point, a very important concept we will explore later.

THE FEEL FULL DIET: *BALANCED*

The Feel Full Diet is based on scientific data gathered in our laboratory at Jefferson Medical College and at other research centers. It is a calorically restricted, *balanced* diet that helps to maximize a feeling of fullness and nutritional satisfaction. Apart from its unique effects in making use of the feel full hormones, effects we've explored in previous chapters, this diet promotes a feeling of satisfaction by providing a balanced mixture of nutrients. This balanced mix is something many weight-loss diets fail to deliver, making for monotonous and ultimately unsatisfying and potentially unhealthy fare.

The Feel Full Diet has all the features necessary for *safe, effective, sustained* weight loss. Balanced, mixed-nutrient diets ensure that you get adequate amounts of essential vitamins and minerals, as well as proper amounts of fat, protein, and carbohydrate. Caloric restriction, moreover, is moderate enough on this diet that you needn't take food supplements or have medical supervision while dieting. (The latter is recommended only if you have some preexisting medical problem such as high blood pressure, diabetes, or high levels of cholesterol and other blood fats—conditions that require medical intervention in any case.) There is growing evidence, moreover, that mixed-nutrient weight-loss diets that allow for 1000 calories or more per day are more sparing of lean body mass. What this means is that a diet like the Feel Full Diet will attack the fat more than it will muscle mass.

THE FEEL FULL DIET: *HEALTHY*

The Feel Full Diet encourages a reduction in cholesterol and saturated fat and an increase in complex carbohydrates and fiber. This is important because the high-fat content of the standard American diet has been implicated as a major risk factor in coronary artery disease (the number one cause of death in men), in breast cancer (the most common form of cancer in women), in colon cancer (the second most frequently occurring cancer in both men and women), and in several other diseases.

Unlike some diets, however, which *insist* upon drastic reductions in fat intake—to such a degree that the dieter quickly gives up and goes back to his or her old way of eating—the Feel Full Diet remains flexible and does not go overboard. I'll show you some easy ways to reduce the fat in your diet without so altering your eating style that you feel deprived.

At the same time I'll show you some easy ways to increase fiber and complex carbohydrate in your diet without feeling as though you've been turned out to graze on the local pasture. I'm certainly mindful of the fat/carbohydrate issue that obsesses so many today, but I'm not neurotic about it. By cutting back on your food intake—something the Feel Full Diet will help you do—you're going to be better off than you were, no matter what you've been eating. Even if you can't change your *relative* intake of fats and carbohydrate, you *can* change your *absolute* intake of these nutrients.

That is, if 40 percent of your calories are derived from fat *before* you begin the Feel Full Diet and if the same percentage of calories still come from fat *after* you've lost weight and gone on our maintenance program, there is no reason to be terribly upset. After all, you will have achieved the primary goal, which is significant caloric reduction, and thus the *absolute* amount of fat you are eating will be reduced significantly, as well. Forty percent of fat from 1200 or even 2000 calories is a very nice improvement over 40 percent of fat from 3000 or 4000 calories or more.

Some argue that the best way to get people to lose weight and change their eating habits permanently is to get them to change the relative proportions of fat, carbohydrate, and protein at the outset and that weight loss will then just naturally follow. I don't agree. The best—and in fact the *only*—way to encourage weight loss is to provide a diet that lets the dieter *feel full*. Once that has happened, the dieter can cut calories and, in so doing, cut back on the absolute amount of fat intake. From that point on—but not before—it is appropriate to make a major point of reordering the relative amounts of fat, protein, and carbohydrates.

This is not to say that I won't *nudge* you in the right direction from the beginning, providing you with information that will enable you to make prudent dietary choices. I *will* do that, and I'll tell you why some choices *are* better than others. Complex carbohydrates and higher-fiber diets, for example, have been shown to help protect against many of the same diseases that high-fat diets promote. They also help promote a feeling of fullness—on fewer calories. They aid digestive regularity and help prevent bowel cancer, diverticulosis, diverticulitis, constipation, hemorrhoids and other varicosities, hiatal hernia, and other conditions. They may also be beneficial in the prevention of gallstones and breast cancer.

I won't, however, *insist* upon radical dietary changes that you can't live with. Such insistence, I'm convinced, would only sabotage our entire effort—which is aimed, first and foremost, at cutting back on the calories.

THE FEEL FULL DIET: *DELICIOUS AND VARIED*

Another of my goals has always been to deliver exciting and varied fare. In Part Two of this book you'll find our meal plans and sample recipes. By skimming ahead to that section now, you'll quickly discover that I'm not sticking you with the sort of diet that tells you "150 ways to make celery hearts scintillating" or "1000 fascinating ways to prepare pineapple for breakfast, lunch, and dinner."

Instead, you'll find such offerings as Brie with Almonds, Quick Beef and Vegetable Soup, Cottage Dip with Crudités, Salmon–Cream Cheese Balls, Viennese Cheese Dumplings, Swiss Steak Dinner with Vegetables, Turkey with Wine and Mushrooms, Creole-Style Fish Dinner, Pasta with Sherried Shrimp, and many more.

THE FEEL FULL DIET: *EFFECTIVE*

Our ultimate goal, of course, is to be effective—that is, to get the pounds off and *keep* them off. The Feel Full Diet is effective because it restricts calories sufficiently to result in steady, significant weight loss. And it *continues* to be effective because it induces a feeling of fullness. Rate of weight loss, of course, will vary from individual to individual, depending upon sex, height, age, present weight, and body build, among other factors. Typically, however, to cite one example, a 150-pound, 5 foot 4 inch, medium-framed, forty-year-old woman could expect the following experience. She is, to begin with, about 30 pounds overweight. Her ideal or target weight (I provide a chart later in the book to help you determine *your* ideal weight) is about 120 pounds. By adhering to the standard Feel Full Diet for women (1200 calories per day), this woman would lose about 2 pounds per week, therefore requiring about four months to reach her goal of 120 pounds. Thereafter she can increase her caloric intake to about 2100 calories per day—the amount typically required to maintain 120 pounds. Again, there is a chart to help you determine your maintenance intake after the weight-loss phase.

A 200-pound, 5 foot 10 inch, medium-framed, twenty-five-year-old man, to cite another typical example, would be about 35 pounds overweight. His target weight is 165 pounds. If he follows the standard Feel Full Diet for men (about 1300 calories per day), he'll lose more than 3 pounds per week, requiring two and a half to three months to arrive at his target. From then on he can consume about 3000 calories per day to maintain his 165 pounds.

The Feel Full Diet is not a crash diet on which you lose ten pounds in four days or thirty pounds in two weeks. Such diets are dangerous and, in the long run, *ineffective*. Any diet that restricts calories will result in some weight loss, and those that restrict calories very sharply will usually result in rapid weight loss. But, as a recent National Institutes of Health consensus committee on obesity reports, fully *90 percent* of all people who lost weight on diets regained *all* of their weight within two years. Some studies indicate that closer to 100 percent of all those who go on crash diets regain all of their weight—and *often more*—usually within a few months.

Thus our goal is slower, steadier, but *permanent* weight loss, typically one to three pounds per week. As discussed in previous chapters, evidence is growing that the base cause of obesity is related to one or more metabolic abnormalities. Just as you would not expect to overwhelm diabetes, also caused by metabolic abnormalities, by treating it with insulin for a few weeks or months, so should you not expect any "quick fix" for the metabolic disorders that result in obesity. Diabetics who adjust to the notion that they must change their *lifelong* behavior to keep their blood sugar under control typically do quite well. By the same token, if you have had long-standing trouble controlling your weight, I can guarantee that you won't overcome your problem as long as you view it as something temporary that can be fixed with another crash diet.

Except in some situations in which there is a temporary disorder creating stress and, in turn, excessive eating, long-term control of weight requires long-term dietary modification. What we really need is gradually to phase out the whole idea of "diet," which to many people implies reduced food intake for a *finite,* relatively short period of time, and substitute instead the concept of "lifestyle change." Most diets are too calorically restricted to be safe for long-term use and/or are too monotonous and unbalanced. The Feel Full Diet, however, is a balanced, mixed-nutrient regimen that offers adequate caloric input to ensure good nutrition. And since it also promotes a feeling of fullness it is ideally suited for long-range weight control. In fact, you could stay on the Feel Full Diet indefinitely without harming yourself.

On now to one of the pleasantest parts of the Feel Full Diet —the satietizer.

6

The Satietizer

SATIETIZER, NOT APPETIZER

HAVE YOU EVER gone to a fancy restaurant anticipating epicurean delights only to return home with half of your main course in a doggy bag? If so, you've probably had this conversation with yourself: "When I went to the restaurant I was really hungry. The servings actually weren't that large, and the food was certainly tasty. So why couldn't I eat it all when I'm able to eat that much at home with no difficulty at all?"

The answer may have to do with what is normally referred to as the "appetizer." An appetizer, as you know, is that generally small premeal morsel that's supposed to put your hunger into high gear just before the entrée arrives, thus making it a pleasure for you to consume the main meal. Well, if an appetizer is composed mainly of carbohydrates and especially if it is eaten just *shortly before* the main meal arrives, it may, indeed, function to stimulate digestive processes that fuel hunger or, as they say, "whet the appetite." If, on the other hand, the appetizer is rich in protein and fat, and if the interval between the premeal and the main course is long enough to permit some emptying of the stomach to occur, then the "appetizer" actually becomes a "satietizer," serving to discourage rather than encourage further food intake.

In other words, if you had Escargots Bernhard, a specialty at the Marquis Restaurant in Denver, as an appetizer, and if your main course, the delightful Rack of Lamb Printaniere with garden-fresh vegetables, didn't arrive until twenty or thirty minutes later, the following would occur. The amino acids in the protein from the snails and the fatty acids from the herb butter and cream would have time to get from the stomach into the first part of the small intestine, where they would stimulate release of some of the fullness hormones. Thus you'd already be experiencing some measure of fullness when your entrée arrived—and half of it could easily end up in the doggy bag for consumption at home later on. Of course, many of us would probably force ourselves to eat the entire course anyway (especially at prevailing prices!), but we wouldn't necessarily enjoy it.

If we're trying to lose weight, nothing helps restrict calories like feeling full. Ideally, it would be nice to have a noncaloric stimulus to release satiety hormones. A drug that could do this is feasible and is, in fact, the object of intense research in my laboratory right now. Human use of such a drug, other than on a very limited, experimental basis, will not occur for some years. At present, the satietizer—a low-calorie premeal enriched with protein, fat, and fiber taken twenty minutes to half an hour before the main course—is the most practical, and pleasant, way to induce earlier-than-normal sensations of fullness.

Fortunately, you don't have to eat Escargots Bernhard to achieve those elusive sensations. Satietizers can be simple—and still very tasty—as you'll see.

WHY THE SATIETIZER IS SAFE AND EFFECTIVE

If you've read the chapters that precede this one you'll already have a pretty good understanding of the mechanisms of hunger and fullness. You're also now familiar with the "fullness hormone," CCK, which is one of several hormones we've studied that affect our eating habits. It was nearly sixty years ago that researchers discovered that dietary fat could stimulate the release of CCK. Other discoveries related to the effects of CCK on the pancreas and gallbladder, both very important in the digestion and metabolism of food, followed. But it was only recently that CCK's ability to stimulate a feeling of fullness began to be understood.

Now we know that CCK is present not only in the small intestine but also in the brain. In fact, specific CCK receptors have now been isolated in certain brain cells. Experiments such as those I have related in preceding chapters make it evident that CCK plays a vital role in sending "satiety signals" to the brain, signals that cause the body to react in ways that create sensations of fullness and thus help discourage further eating.

And where it all starts is with fat and protein. These nutrients, once they reach the small intestine, cause the body to release CCK (and other hormones). These hormones, in turn, "communicate" with the brain to produce satiety.

The Feel Full Diet is the first eating program to use these new discoveries in the construction of a safe and balanced diet. There have been other very well-known high-fat or high-protein diets in the past which unwittingly manipulated the fullness hormones. I say "unwittingly" because the people who constructed those diets knew nothing about CCK. Some of those high-fat and high-protein diets were effective in helping people lose weight—but the diets were unbalanced and were validly criticized by many as unhealthy. Equally bad, they were monotonous, and people couldn't stand to stay on them for very long. Most gained back all the weight they had lost.

The Feel Full Diet, on the other hand, puts the fat and protein where it can do the most good—*before* the main meal in the form of the satietizer. The satietizer, in a sense, is an expression of dietary "fine tuning." Instead of hitting the body with massive amounts of fat and protein, as some earlier diet authors recommended, the Feel Full Diet works—and far more effectively—with relatively small amounts of fat and protein by strategically introducing them "up front."

The satietizers *are* mostly fat and protein, but each satietizer is small, only 150 to 200 calories. This fat and protein in the premeal satietizer delivers adequate amounts of these CCK-stimulating substances into the small intestine well before the lower-fat, lower-protein main course is started. This strategy allows the intestinal phase of satiety or fullness (explained in Chapter 1) to be activated early enough to discourage overeating.

Total intake of fat on this diet—30 to 35 percent—is actually lower than the present average American intake of 40 to 45 percent, and the feel full mechanisms will still work. Thirty to 35 percent of calories from fat is exactly what the American Heart Association recommends as the healthy maximum. And the actual, absolute reduction in fat on the Feel Full Diet is actually much greater. For instance, if you normally eat 2500 calories per day and 40 percent of that is fat, on the Feel Full Diet you'll eat 1250 calories per day and reduce fat intake from 111 grams to 49 grams per day. That represents a 56 percent total reduction in fat intake.

The approximate percentage of protein in the Feel Full Diet is 12 to 15 percent, consistent with American Heart Association guidelines. That leaves about 50 percent of the calories in the form of carbohydrates.

Although the overall diet, *including* satietizers, is about 35 percent fat, 15 percent protein, and 50 percent carbohydrate, in the satietizers themselves about 55 percent of the calories, sometimes less and sometimes more, are in the form of fat and protein. For instance, an eight-ounce serving of cream of broccoli soup used as a satietizer provides 140 calories, of which *40 percent are fat*, 13 percent protein, and 47 percent carbohydrate. An eight-ounce serving of plain low-fat yogurt used as an "emergency satietizer" has 150 calories, of which 24 percent are fat, *31 percent protein*, and 45 percent carbohydrates.

SATIETIZERS: SIMPLE TO GOURMET

As stated earlier, satietizers don't have to be elaborate. You'll find a number of them in Part Two of this book that are very simple and even highly portable, meaning you can carry them with you and eat them at your desk before going out to lunch. This is important, I've found, particularly when you consider how little time many people who work have these days (and that is true for people who work in the home, too). Many of our satietizers can be made up in large batches and then refrigerated or frozen for future use.

To give you an idea of what one of our simpler but very popular satietizers is like, consider our Peanut Butter–Honey Balls. To make four "A" or three "B" servings ("A" servings are 150 calories and are for women; "B" servings are 200 calories and are for men), here's all you need: ⅓ cup instant nonfat dry milk powder; 4½ tablespoons smooth or crunchy peanut butter; 1½ tablespoons honey; and 1½ tablespoons unsweetened cocoa (or additional milk powder if you don't like chocolate).

Combine the first three ingredients in a medium-sized bowl. Mix well with a spoon to form a pliable dough that is neither crumbly nor sticky. If the mixture is very dry, add water, drop by drop, until it is the right consistency. If it is too sticky, add a few pinches of milk powder. Form the mixture into 12 equal-sized balls (or roll it into a 12-inch log and cut into 1-inch slices). Coat each ball (or slice) with the cocoa or additional milk powder. These can be stored in an airtight container in the refrigerator for two weeks or longer. One "A" serving equals three Peanut Butter–Honey Balls. One "B" serving equals four of the balls.

Here's another example, drawn from some of our more elaborate satietizers (even these, though, aren't at all difficult or particularly time-consuming, and they're great for guests, too): Viennese Cheese Dumplings. For this tasty concoction, you'll need one 12-ounce container of dry-curd cottage cheese; 1 large egg yolk; 2½ tablespoons of dry Cream of Rice cereal or Cream of Wheat cereal; 1 tablespoon sugar; 1 teaspoon lemon juice; ¼ cup fine crushed corn flake crumbs; and (optional) unsweetened applesauce and ground cinnamon.

You can mash the cottage cheese with a fork or put it through a sieve if the curds are large or you prefer a smoother dumpling. Stir in the egg yolk, cereal, sugar, and lemon juice. Let the mixture stand for about five minutes.

Next put the corn flake crumbs in a small bowl. Divide the cheese mixture into twelve equal portions. One at a time, spoon each portion into the crumbs; then coat it with the crumbs and use your hands to form a ball. Place the balls on a nonstick spray-coated baking sheet. Bake in a preheated 350° F oven for about twenty minutes or until quite firm. Serve the balls warm, at room temperature, or chilled. If desired, top each ball with 1 teaspoon applesauce and a pinch of cinnamon. One "A" serving equals three balls. One "B" serving equals four balls. This recipe will make four "A" or three "B" servings.

I recommend that a noncaloric or very low caloric beverage be consumed along with the satietizer. Water is ideal. If you find water too dull, you might try mineral water with a little lime or lemon. Coffee or iced tea *with artificial sweetener only* or diet soda can also be used. Take eight to twelve ounces of one of these liquids with your satietizer. This will help promote gastric emptying and add to the feeling of fullness.

Alcohol contains a lot of calories and should not be used *with* the satietizer. Alcohol has variable effects on appetite and satiety in different individuals. Some of my patients are accustomed to having a drink or two before dinner and wonder how it will affect their diet. I tell them that alcohol is not magically exempted from caloric restrictions. It's amazing how many people go on diets, religiously count every calorie consumed during each of three meals, but then completely ignore calories consumed in the form of "extras,"—snacks, drinks, nibbles—all of which can add up monumentally. I've encountered a number of individuals, in fact, who regularly consume more in "extras" each day than they do during their three regular meals.

Now you may have noticed that I said alcohol should not be used *with* the satietizer. In some cases it is permissible to use it *in place of* or as an alternate form of satietizer. Unfortunately, it is only through trial and error that you can determine whether one alcoholic drink (not exceeding 150 to 200 calories) will work well for you. Overall, I don't find that alcohol works nearly as well as our standard satietizer, but in some individuals a glass of wine or beer as a satietizer may work nicely.

Here, to help you stay within caloric guidelines, are the caloric contents of some typical alcoholic beverages:

12-ounce can or bottle of beer—150 calories
3½-ounce glass of wine (average)—87 calories
1 ounce of scotch or other hard liquor (average)—65 calories

Remember that if you add other items to mixed drinks, such as cream, you will increase the caloric content of those drinks dramatically. *All* calories count—*equally.*

While on the subject of snacking, I'd like to make a happy observation. A number of my patients have noted that the satietizer has helped them not only eat less during their main meals but also has helped them cut back on snacks. I'm not sure exactly why this is; perhaps it's that the satietizer seems like a snack in itself—and since it seems like a rich one in most cases it may have psychological "holding power." One woman called the satietizer a "guiltless snack." She used to start snacking the minute she got home. She still does that—but with *one* satietizer. Then she gets her dinner ready quickly and eats it about twenty or thirty minutes later, observing the intrameal interval and timing procedure I'll say more about in the next chapter.

Another woman put it this way: "I used to snack all the time without even thinking about it. At the end of the day I couldn't possibly have told you everything I'd snacked on throughout the day. Now I know I can have those two satietizers, which I think of as snacks, and that keeps me focused on what I'm eating. It hasn't been nearly as difficult as I imagined to give up on all those extras."

"EMERGENCY" SATIETIZERS—A BAKER'S DOZEN

One of the best ways to avoid compulsive snacking is always to have satietizers on hand. That way you can't say, "Well, I'm out of satietizers today, so I'll just have a few snacks instead." As I've already pointed out, satietizers can be very simple or they can be gourmet-quality selections. Here are a "baker's dozen" satietizers you can use in emergencies, or on a regular basis, whenever you have failed to prepare the ordinary satietizers. These will work just as well. But remember, the same rule applies here—just *one* satietizer twenty minutes before lunch and another twenty minutes before dinner. (We've found that satietizers before breakfast aren't usually necessary; it's at lunch and dinner that most people overeat. I'll have more to say about breakfasts later on in this book.)

The quantities inside parentheses are "B" quantities for men, providing 200 instead of 150 calories.

1. 1½ tablespoons (2 tablespoons) peanut butter spread inside celery sticks
2. 1 (1⅓) cooked frankfurter(s) (hot dogs), cut into slices and dipped in mustard (Tip: Eat with a toothpick; it takes longer.)
3. 1½ ounces (2 ounces) luncheon meat spread lightly with mustard or horseradish and rolled inside a large lettuce leaf

4. 2 ounces (3 ounces) sliced cooked chicken breast, turkey breast, or turkey pastrami, eaten on one slice of whole wheat or rye bread

5. 3 ounces (4 ounces) canned water-packed tuna or canned white meat chicken mixed with 1 tablespoon (1½ tablespoons) reduced-calorie mayonnaise or similar dressing

6. 2 ounces (3 ounces) canned chunk chicken (light and dark) mixed with 1 tablespoon (1½ tablespoons) reduced-calorie mayonnaise or similar dressing

7. 6 ounces (1 cup) vanilla or coffee low-fat yogurt

8. 2 ounces (3 ounces) part-skim mozzarella cheese, cut into cubes and eaten with a toothpick (see #2)

9. 1 ounce (1½ ounces) luncheon meat rolled around ¾ ounce (1 ounce) thinly sliced part-skim mozzarella cheese

10. 1 hard-boiled egg mashed with 1 tablespoon (1½ tablespoons) reduced-calorie mayonnaise or similar dressing and served on a tomato half

11. ¾ cup (1 cup) low-fat cottage cheese topped with 2 tablespoons unsweetened applesauce

12. 2 ounces (3 ounces) sardines canned in tomato or mustard sauce with 3 (4) saltine crackers

13. 1½ ounces (2 ounces) mozzarella or American cheese melted on a rice "cake" cracker in a microwave or toaster oven (may be sprinkled with dried herbs)

Many canned soups can also serve nicely as emergency or quickie satietizers. Various studies have attested to the ability of some soups to fill people up faster than many other foods of equal calories. Here are a few examples of soups you might consider using as satietizers:

1. Cream of mushroom soup, 6-ounce serving, 150 calories
2. Sirloin burger chunky soup, 6-ounce serving, 140 calories
3. Creamy broccoli soup, 4-ounce serving, 140 calories
4. Chicken noodle soup, 6-ounce serving, 140 calories

For people who like to munch on potato chips and nachos but

end up eating too many calories, Spicer's Nutriwheat™ is a great substitute. At 110 calories a bag, this product is high in protein as well as fiber and makes a very good satietizer. (It is available in multiple flavors including sour cream and onion and barbecue.) Spicer's Nutriwheat can be eaten alone or mixed with one-third cup of plain yogurt (total 160 calories). This product is not available in food stores but can be ordered by calling 800-824-3196. In addition to these emergency satietizers, you'll find thirty-six of our thoroughly tested "regular" satietizers in Part Two of this book.

SUMMING UP: SATISFACTION GUARANTEED?

Remember, the satietizer is a small premeal course that is richer in fat and/or protein than the main course. It is designed to stimulate release of the feel full hormones at a strategic time. This strategy requires that you consume your satietizer *twenty minutes before* you eat your main meal. Drink eight to twelve ounces of water or diet beverage with your satietizer.

Will this *guarantee* that you won't feel as hungry as you have in the past? No. In the diet world *nothing* is guaranteed, no matter what anybody tells you. Nonetheless, on the basis of the best available evidence and the experience of my patients, I believe the concept of the satietizer to be of crucial importance in curbing hunger—the biochemically mediated sensation that, more than psychology, stress, or anything else, keeps people eating long after they should have stopped.

The satietizer is only part of the picture, although a very important part. Don't start your diet program until you have read the rest of this book carefully. Next we'll consider the importance of timing, the *intra*meal interval, and the *inter*meal interval. The Feel Full Diet is as concerned with *when you eat* as it is with *what you eat.*

7

When You Eat Is as
Important as *What* You Eat

THE TIMING FACTORS

MOST DIETS FOCUS entirely on *what* to eat and *how much* to
eat. But our research has convinced us that just as important is
the issue of *when* to eat. The correct timing of food intake is
very important in reducing that intake. Timing involves several
factors:

1. Number of meals per day
2. Amount of time spent consuming each meal
3. The *intra*meal interval
4. The *inter*meal interval

The *intra*meal interval is the space of time *within* each individual lunch or dinner that separates satietizer from main
course. The *inter*meal interval is the amount of time between
the main meals.

Let's consider each of these factors in turn.

You have probably read about diets that encourage you to eat several small meals per day instead of the standard three. Various theories have been put forward in support of these recommendations, but the theories have not been accompanied by scientific evidence. I won't bandy words. I prefer sticking with the traditional number of meals consumed each day. The Feel Full Diet works best with the standard three—or standard two and a half (since many people don't make much of a production out of breakfast). And from what I have observed, you are likely to eat less if you eat three meals a day. I've seen too many people who were encouraged to "eat when you feel like it" eating all the time, drifting from one snack to the next every waking hour.

The standard three meals make very good sense. First, it's logical to refuel, to break the fast of sleep, upon awakening. Even a light breakfast will usually get you on your way and will buffer the acidic environment that builds up overnight. In people who have hyperacidity or stress or are prone to peptic ulcer disease, early morning can be a time of gastric rumblings or even pain, which is relieved by eating. Then, from both a digestive and an energy-demand point of view, it is logical to have another meal four to six hours later. Lunch gets us through the rest of the day to evening, when, again, the digestive and metabolic processes are ideally suited for more food. Dinner usually follows lunch by five to seven hours.

Another good reason for sticking to the standard three regimen has to do with sleep. If we eat too close to the time we go to bed (which could be one consequence of eating several small meals per day), problems often result, making it difficult to fall asleep or stay asleep. Any "heaviness" that we experience as a result of eating is often accentuated when we lie down or become completely inactive. In addition, acid secretion from the stomach is stimulated between one and three hours after a meal, and this can cause heartburn and other symptoms of dyspepsia during attempted sleep. This is because acid reflux into the esophagus (heartburn) can occur more easily in the reclining position.

Apart from all this, nibbling away at food whenever you feel like it makes it difficult to harness the "feel full" mechanisms we've been discussing. If we want those signals of fullness to reach the brain loud and clear, we need to keep the channels open. You might think of those snacks and little meals squeezed in here and there willy-nilly throughout the day as "noise" that gets in the way of satiety signals.

So three meals a day is the way to go. This regimen is easier on your stomach and makes it easier for you to keep track of exactly how many calories you're consuming. Most important, it makes it easier for the feel full signals to do their work effectively.

AMOUNT OF TIME SPENT CONSUMING EACH MEAL

The length of each meal is a complex but very important issue. Typically people sit down and eat until full in one great "nosh"—or at least too fast to permit the feel full hormonal mechanisms to "kick in." Researchers have shown that *at least* 650 calories are easily consumed in a typical twenty-minute burst of eating that approximates the standard meal. If we introduce the feel full hormone CCK into the bloodstream of the typical person while consuming that meal, fullness occurs earlier, and it is possible to consume far fewer calories before feeling satisfied.

Unfortunately, it is not practical to give the millions of overweight people in this country intravenous CCK—and it is ineffective when given orally. (This, as noted earlier, has not stopped the unscrupulous from marketing products that are falsely claimed to contain CCK.) We must rely on methods that can stimulate *the body's own* CCK—which is what the Feel Full

Diet does. The best way to do this is to lengthen the time of the meal, starting with the satietizer, followed by the twenty-minute *intra*meal interval during which no further food is eaten, and concluding with the main course. This strategy lengthens the period of time during which food is consumed, allows CCK and other hormones to start working, and reduces total caloric intake.

We've found that by lengthening the meal to about forty to fifty minutes we can match the effects of the intravenous CCK. This is done by using a satietizer, which usually takes no more than ten minutes to eat (we encourage eating the satietizers at a leisurely pace, savoring them), observing a twenty-minute *intra*meal interval, and then eating a small main course. Thus, what might have been a meal of at least 650 calories is reduced to a meal of about 450 calories.

THE *INTRA*MEAL INTERVAL

Let's look more closely at the *intra*meal interval. "Intra" means within. This is the space of time between the satietizer and the main meal. What is the rationale for that twenty-minute space of time, and what are you supposed to do during that time period?

The concentration of CCK in the blood during fasting periods is so small it can't be measured in most laboratories. But those labs with sensitive enough assays can show that within twenty minutes of beginning a meal CCK concentrations increase by two and a half times to near maximal levels. Even at peak levels, CCK is present in the bloodstream only in incredibly minute quantities. But CCK is like other peptide hormones, such as insulin and growth hormone, in being able to control highly complex biochemical events in the body at very low concentrations. CCK is very potent stuff.

The typical, *non*-feel full meal usually takes no more than twenty minutes to consume. It ends at that point in part because by then there is enough CCK in the bloodstream to signal satiety. As many a cook who has spent hours preparing a meal only to see it gobbled down in minutes will attest, this twenty-minute estimate for the typical meal is probably on the long side. Most people can put away formidable numbers of calories before the fullness signals are sent to the brain. Those signals start going out loud and clear about twenty minutes after a meal is started, especially if there is ample fat and protein in the meal, and then they persist for some time thereafter.

The key to cutting calories, then, is very clearly to limit food intake during the first twenty to thirty minutes before the CCK signals start to work. Eating very slowly may help accomplish this, but many people have trouble eating slowly. Our solution is to eat the satietizer followed by a twenty-minute wait before starting the main course. The satietizer should be consumed slowly. Nibble at it, if possible, over a five- or ten-minute period. But even if you gobble it right down it will still do its work—which is to set in motion the feel full mechanisms. Then wait twenty minutes and eat your main meal. By the time you start the main meal, CCK and other hormones will be at work and you will find the smaller-than-normal entrée far more filling than otherwise.

What should you do during that twenty-minute intrameal interval? Well, first of all, twenty minutes isn't a particularly long time. And as we've seen, satietizers aren't elaborate productions that need to be spread across the dining room table. You can enjoy your satietizer, and accompanying beverage, while starting preparations for the main meal for yourself and/or the rest of the family. You can have your satietizer and then watch the early evening news. You can eat it at your desk before lunch, timing it so you'll arrive at the restaurant and be eating your main course twenty to thirty minutes later. Or you can read, talk on the phone, or do any number of household or take-home tasks during that brief period. Some people prefer to do nothing.

One woman said, "I find that time period very good for meditating or just thinking about things other than food. Or if I do think about food, I think about how good the satietizer was and how much better it is to be exerting some control over my eating habits rather than just letting food rule my life."

That word "control" has been mentioned by several of my patients. The Feel Full Diet, they say, gives them a sense of participation, of doing something, actively and logically, that they felt was lacking in many of the other diets they tried. The twenty-minute intrameal interval becomes a symbol of that control—a period during which it is not only possible but pleasant *not* to eat.

It *is* permissible to drink more water or *diet* beverage (as much as you like) during the twenty-minute interval. It is also permissible to engage in light exercise during the interval. A twenty-minute walk not only fills up the time but burns calories and, in many people, further dampens appetite. (For more details on exercise, see Chapter 12.)

THE *INTER*MEAL INTERVAL

Once a meal is finished there is a period of time before hunger is experienced again and a new meal is started. This period is called the *inter*meal interval. I raise this subject only because most animal studies show that the smaller a meal is, the shorter the intermeal interval. In other words, if you eat a small amount, it won't be long before you eat again. In a sense, this is just another way of looking at the issues related to number of meals per day, which I've already discussed. Numerous small meals per day may, as I've pointed out, actually lead to greater, not lesser, caloric intake than having "three squares" per day.

But since the main meals (see the next chapter) in the Feel Full Diet are relatively small, you may wonder if this won't lead to shorter intermeal intervals—to a more rapid return of hunger. We have not found this to be the case. One probable reason is that although the Feel Full meals are reduced in calories they are eaten over a significantly longer period of time than are standard meals. This "stretching out" of the meal may also lengthen the period of time during which CCK levels remain elevated after the meal is completed. In addition, psychological factors related to longer meals may tend to reduce the need to eat again as soon as might be the case with a standard meal.

THE STRATEGY SO FAR

All of this might seem quite complex, and in some ways it is. But this chapter, I hope, has enabled you to appreciate that successful dieting has a lot to do with factors that usually are ignored—number of meals consumed daily, length of meals, time intervals between meals, and our unique time interval *within* the meal between the satietizer and main course.

In practice it's all really quite simple:

1. Stick to the standard three meals per day (modifications with respect to breakfast are permitted, as explained in the next chapter).

2. Eat a satietizer approximately twenty minutes before eating lunch and another satietizer twenty minutes before dinner. Drink water or a diet beverage with your satietizer, as explained in the preceding chapter. Spend five to ten minutes, if possible, nibbling on your satietizer.

3. Wait twenty minutes after you finish your satietizer before starting your main course. Do not eat anything during this twenty-minute intrameal interval. You may, however, have more water or diet beverage during the twenty-minute interval.

4. Proceed to the main course at the conclusion of the twenty minutes.

8

The Main Course

LOTS OF FOODS TO CHOOSE FROM

IF YOU'LL SKIP ahead for a moment to Chapter 13 in Part Two (The Fourteen-Day Feel Full Menu Plan), you'll quickly grasp just how varied this diet can be. Or simply skim over the foods listed in the Table of Contents of Part Two. Under Main Dishes, you'll find recipes for a number of different food categories: Meat, Poultry, Fish and Shellfish, Vegetarian, Side Dishes and Quick Breads, Breakfast Dishes, and Desserts.

Swiss Steak Dinner with Vegetables, Chili con Carne, Curried Beef, Chick-Peas and Cauliflower, Chicken in Orange Sauce, Chicken Cacciatore, Turkey Normandy, Creole-Style Fish Dinner, Hearty New England–Style Fish Chowder, Linguine with White Scallop Sauce, Zucchini Lasagne, Easy Ratatouille, Acorn Squash Stuffed with Apples, Raisin-Bran Muffins, Whole Wheat Irish Soda Bread, Mock Cheese Danish, Dutch Apple Pancakes, Strawberry and Cheese Crêpes, Easiest Ever Raspberry Sherbet, Piña Colada Chiffon Squares, and Frozen Banana Fudgies are just a few of the fabulous foods available to you for main course and dessert fare.

CONSTRUCTING THE MAIN COURSE

Our Fourteen-Day Feel Full Menu Plan in Chapter 13 will give you many ideas about how you might compose your main meals. Remember, if you are a woman you will be eating two satietizers each day—one before lunch and one before dinner. These will be 150 calories each. That means you'll get 300 of your 1200 calories from satietizers each day, leaving 900 calories to be derived from other foods. If you're a man, you'll also be eating two satietizers per day, each 200 calories for a total of 400 calories from that source. That will leave 900 calories (for a total of 1300) to be obtained from other foods.

By studying the recipes in Part Two, each of which comes with full information about the caloric content of all ingredients (the figures are in brackets following the name of the ingredient) and each serving, you can easily construct meals that add up to the prescribed number of calories—approximately 900 not counting the satietizers. As you study the recipes in Part Two, note that almost all of them make more than one serving. The extra servings can either be reserved for other meals or served to other members of the family. Unlike the recipes used in so many other weight-loss programs, ours are suitable for everyone. Naturally, you must take care to divide the recipes into *equal* servings to ensure that you—the dieter—do not exceed the caloric limits I've prescribed.

All of our recipes have been designed to be easy on the palate. They do not depart radically from standard American fare yet manage to reduce the total amount of fat, and especially saturated fat, in the diet while, at the same time, increasing intake of complex carbohydrates and fiber. Complex carbohydrates (see the discussion below) are *not,* contrary to the common assumption, fattening.

Overall, I like to see my patients reduce their relative fat intake 5 to 10 percent, or even more if they can tolerate it. You should strive to obtain no more than 30 to 35 percent of your calories from fat, about 15 percent from protein, and the rest (50 to 55 percent) from carbohydrates. You don't have to make a fetish out of this, checking to see where every calorie is coming from. You can make considerable progress in the right direction by making fairly simple modifications in your diet. Most of you are already getting about 15 percent of all your calories from protein. That doesn't have to change. All you have to concentrate on is cutting back on fat and increasing carbohydrate and fiber.

TIPS ON CUTTING THE FAT

As you progress through the weight-loss phase of the Feel Full Diet, you can speed your progress and make the weight-maintenance phase easier if you'll practice some of the following with respect to your main courses:

• Trim all visible fat from meat and remove the skin from poultry before baking, broiling, roasting, or stewing. Use a rack to drain off excess fat whenever possible. Avoid *frying* foods as much as possible.

• Use vegetable oils (of the polyunsaturated variety) in place of animal fats (such as butter) in your cooking. But remember, vegetable fats are also loaded with calories. Using soft or liquid margarines in place of butter will eliminate a lot of fat, cholesterol, and calories.

• Cut back on *all* fats, especially animal fats.

• Cut back on your egg consumption. Eggs are freighted with fat and cholesterol, both of which have been implicated in heart disease and other serious disorders. If a recipe calls for an egg yolk, substitute *two* egg whites instead. You'll be amazed at how well this works in most baked goods. Some recipes in the

Feel Full Diet do use whole eggs when the total fat content of the recipe can be held to an acceptable level.

• Not all cheeses are created equal. Some are quite a bit lower in fat than others. Supermarkets are, increasingly, carrying "reduced-calorie" and "diet" cheeses. Try them. Many are quite tasty. Low-fat cottage cheeses, ricotta cheese, and part-skim mozzarella cheese are good choices for cooking. Cheddar, by the way, is one of the highest-fat cheeses.

• Eat less red meat and more fish and poultry (skinned). Both chicken and turkey are much lower in fat than beef, pork, lamb, and such meats. Fish is a particularly good choice because it contains a special class of fatty acids that have recently been shown to reduce cholesterol levels.

• *Sample* desserts, if you can't go without, but don't eat the whole thing. Most desserts contain a lot of fat.

• Reduce intake of nuts, all of which are very high in fat. So are sunflower seeds.

• Use diet salad dressings and imitation mayonnaise and mock sour cream instead of the real thing. When you order a salad in a restaurant, ask for the dressing on the side. Then use it, if at all, sparingly.

• If you eat a lot of hamburger, buy the lean or extra-lean variety in the supermarket.

TIPS ON INCREASING INTAKE OF COMPLEX CARBOHYDRATES AND FIBER

• In general, try to replace the fat you're eliminating from your diet with fruits, vegetables, bread, pasta, legumes, rice, and other grain and cereal dishes. These are rich in complex carbohydrates and fiber. Bread and pasta are not necessarily fattening, and carbohydrates are loaded with health-giving vitamins, minerals, and other nutrients.

• Try to eat fresh fruit and vegetables at least once a day. Eat these whole and/or in salads. Steamed or canned vegetables are also good choices. Whenever possible, avoid canned fruits because they usually come in thick, calorie-laden syrup. If canned fruit is to be used, drain off the syrup and make sure that the caloric value of the syrup is taken into account when adding up your calories.

• Experiment with different breads. Whole wheat, bran, oat bread, and others in which the grains have not been overly refined deliver the most fiber and complex carbohydrate. Be aware, however, that many of the so-called "health food" breads have a lot of sugar and refined sugar in them.

• Try cooked cereal for a change. Oats, wheat, and mixed grains all are excellent cereal choices.

• Increase your intake of beans, peas, and other legumes. If you like Mexican food, indulge—but watch out for excess fat in some restaurant offerings. Beans, tacos, and the like are great sources of complex carbohydrate—and, again, they are *not* fattening.

• Try pasta dishes—spaghetti, linguine, and the like. Italian food is wonderful—so long as you watch the sauces. The red sauces are best. The white sauces tend to be high in fat.

• If you have to snack, try to get away from fatty snacks and get into carbohydrates instead. Popcorn, without butter (a little margarine is okay), is an excellent choice. Carrot sticks, fruit, whole wheat melba toasts, and low-fat crackers are all good snack choices.

These are just tips, not rules. During the weight-loss phase of your diet you'll make progress as long as you stick to the caloric guidelines. But you'll make even faster progress if you follow some of these tips. (If you decide to get serious about the low-fat, high-carbohydrate way of eating, there are many good books on this subject. Perhaps the best is *The New American Diet* by Sonja Connor and William Connor, M.D., the people who pioneered the low-fat/high-carbohydrate diet.)

Until you've lost the weight you want to shed you will probably stick mostly to the recipes in this book. Later, when you enter the weight-maintenance phase, you'll undoubtedly expand your dietary repertoire. At the back of the book you will find an extensive chart that lists the fat, protein, carbohydrate, fiber, and calorie contents of dozens of foods to help keep you on the right track. You can run a spot-check from time to time to see how much of your diet is composed of fats, proteins, and carbohydrates.

SUMMARY

After eating your satietizer (150 calories for women, 200 calories for men), wait twenty minutes (during which time you may drink water or diet beverages but may not eat anything) and then begin your main course. Main courses must not exceed 900 calories *per day total* on the standard weight-loss program (for alternatives, see the next two chapters). You may distribute these 900 calories as you see fit, but, as pointed out earlier, I strongly recommend spreading them across the three meals. *Generally* what works best is a small breakfast (around 200 calories) and lunches and dinners in which the main meal accounts for about 350 calories each.

Follow the sample menus or selected dishes from the recipes in Part Two to construct your own meal plans. Strive to reduce fat intake while increasing complex carbohydrate intake (breads, grains, cereals, beans, peas, fruits, and vegetables).

Eat slowly. Try to spend about twenty minutes eating your main course. Don't consider yourself a failure, however, if you eat more quickly than that. The main thing is to stay within the caloric boundaries, which is easier to do on this diet than on most, thanks to the satietizer, the mixed nature of the fare, and the other timing elements I discussed earlier.

Remember that the Feel Full Diet has two separate stages— the premeal satietizer and the main course. Different rules apply to the two different stages. Satietizers are high in fat and protein because these nutrients, introduced in small quantities at the appropriate time, stimulate CCK. So we encourage (though, again, only in *small,* but concentrated, quantities) fat and protein in the first stage and then cutting down on those nutrients during the second stage. By the same token, we discourage carbohydrates during the first stage (because they do not promote a feeling of fullness at that point) and encourage them during the second stage. So don't eat bread *before* the main course— stick to the prescribed satietizers. Save the bread and other carbohydrates for the main meal.

Now on to a couple of variations on the "standard" weight-loss program—one for women who want to lose weight faster than on the 1200-calorie program and one for men who find 1300 calories per day too restrictive.

9

Optional Faster Weight Loss for Women

SHOULD *YOU* GO FOR FASTER WEIGHT LOSS?

AS I'VE STRESSED several times, *gradual* but steady weight loss is preferable to very fast, sudden weight loss. I've already pointed out the pitfalls of crash diets. Diets that offer 800 calories per day or less are, in my view, unwise and should definitely be avoided. Nonetheless, there are some women for whom a 1000-calorie-per-day diet is suitable. I consider women in the following categories candidates for this optional 1000-calorie diet;

1. Women who are *very* motivated to lose weight at a faster rate. There are some individuals who do not *remain* motivated unless they see relatively rapid progress. Again, however, I would caution you not to go overboard. *Under no circumstances should you consume fewer than 1000 calories*

per day unless specifically instructed to do so by a qualified medical doctor.

2. Women who find the standard 1200-calorie Feel Full Diet *too* filling. Believe it or not, hungry as you no doubt are even as you read this, there *are* women who have had this experience.

3. Women who do not lose weight after strictly adhering to the standard 1200-calorie diet for at least one month. Some, especially those who have tried many diets in the past and have always regained weight, are likely to have a metabolic set point problem that makes it particularly difficult to lose weight. Such women generally need to combine caloric restriction with a program of exercise so as to "reset" the set point. For further details, see Chapter 12, related to exercise, diet, and set point.

VITAMIN/MINERAL SUPPLEMENTATION

It is essential to take vitamin/mineral supplementation with 1000-calorie (and less) diets. Take a good quality "one-a-day" or "insurance formula" to get adequate micronutrition. Many vitamin/mineral products are poorly balanced, so you must be careful what you buy. If you decide to go for the "one-a-day" approach, the Centrum High Potency Multivitamin/Multimineral Formula from Lederle Laboratories (available without prescription in most drugstores and many supermarkets) is one of the few I can recommend. This Centrum preparation will provide women with enough of all the important micronutrients, including iron, with the exception of calcium. You can buy calcium supplements in any health-food store or drugstore and in many larger grocery stores. Calcium *carbonate* is the best form in which to buy calcium. Supplement your diet with 500 to 1000 milligrams (one gram) of calcium daily.

The best "insurance formula" I've found is one you can order by mail, and it is a particularly good value. It is called Broad

Spectrum, and it is available from NutriGuard Research (write to P.O. Box 865, Encinitas, California 92024 for an order form). Broad Spectrum provides a superb balance of vitamins and minerals and contains 1000 milligrams of calcium in the form of calcium carbonate so that you don't need an extra calcium supplement. "Insurance formulas" are those that cover all micronutrient needs, except in special cases. They are ideal for dieters.

While on this subject, let me add that even those on the standard 1200-calorie Feel Full Diet—or *any* weight-loss diet—can benefit from a good one-a-day or insurance formula. I recommend it. But it's absolutely essential on 1000-calorie-or-less diets.

It's best to take your vitamin/mineral supplements just after meals.

CONSTRUCTION OF THE 1000-CALORIE DIET

Again, you can distribute the 1000 calories as you see fit, but I still recommend three meals a day. Generally, what I find works best is the following regimen:

> 200 calories breakfast
> 150 calories prelunch satietizer
> 200 calories lunch main meal
> 150 calories predinner satietizer
> 300 calories dinner main meal
> ———————
> 1000 calories total

This distribution of calories is just a suggestion. Some variations will do no harm as long as you stick to a total of 1000 calories. From the recipes in Part Two you will be able to construct many variations adding up to 1000 calories per day. You can also make the Fourteen-Day Feel Full Menu Plan in Part

Two work for you. You just have to knock off 200 calories from those menus each day. Your satietizers, however, should always remain at 150 calories. You can change the caloric content of servings (listed at the end of each recipe) by increasing the number of servings per recipe. For example, if you find a recipe that makes four servings at 250 calories per serving, you can divide the recipe into five servings instead. Then each serving will be only 200 calories. For additional help, consult the calorie chart at the end of the book.

10

Optional Higher-Calorie Program for Men

WHICH MEN NEED THE HIGHER-CALORIE PROGRAM?

SOME MEN FIND the standard 1300-calorie diet too restrictive. These men lose weight quickly on the standard regimen but find that they are sometimes still hungry. For these men we recommend an 1800-calorie-per-day program. Many of them still are able to lose one to three pounds per week. Who are these men?

1. Men over 5 feet 10 inches tall.

2. Men who consume more than 3000 calories per day before starting the diet.

3. Any man who finds he is still hungry after trying the standard Feel Full Diet for at least a few days.

CONSTRUCTION OF THE 1800-CALORIE DIET

I recommend a distribution of calories for each day approximately as follows:

> 400 calories breakfast
> 200 calories prelunch satietizer
> 400 calories lunch main meal
> 200 calories predinner satietizer
> 400 calories dinner main meal
> 200 calories dessert
>
> _____
>
> 1800 calories total

Again, this is just a suggestion. Use the recipes in Part Two and the calorie chart at the end of the book to make combinations not exceeding 1800 calories per day. Do not alter the satietizers. Those must remain at 200 calories. You'll find dessert recipes in Part Two.

11

Weight Maintenance
(After Weight Loss)

HOW MUCH *SHOULD* YOU WEIGH?

THERE CONTINUES TO be a controversy over what "ideal" body weights should be for different individuals of different ages, sexes, body build, and activity levels. Weight charts you've probably seen tend to be quite permissive in the view of many experts on obesity. That is, they tend to say, in effect, that it's okay to gain weight as you age. There is, in fact, a natural tendency to gain as we get older—in part because we become more sedentary.

Some authorities believe that if you were healthy and considered yourself well-proportioned when you were about twenty years of age, your weight at that stage in your life was and *still is* probably close to being "ideal" for you. The idea that it's okay to gain between twenty and forty pounds between ages twenty and fifty, as so commonly happens, is faulty, these authorities say. As we age, our muscle and bone masses diminish, making us less, not more, able comfortably and healthily to carry extra weight. And, of course, some people gain far more than twenty to forty pounds, putting an even heavier burden on a body increasingly less sturdy.

It's also possible, of course, to go overboard. "Ideals" are not always realistic. Life is typically far from ideal in many particulars. I ask my patients to use the 1983 Metropolitan Height and Weight Tables at the back of the book (page 216) to get some idea of what they should weigh. I prefer to think of "target weight" or "goal weight" rather than ideal weight. Let's say you are a 5 foot 5 inch woman of medium build who now weighs 170 pounds. Nobody has to tell you you're overweight. But you may be confused about how much weight you really need to lose.

Consult the Height and Weight Tables and you'll see that the "average" weight for a woman of your height is 134 pounds. This is derived from an average range of 127 to 141 pounds. The average weight—134 pounds—is probably close to the "ideal" for a woman of your height. It may or may not be realistic for you to aim for that weight. If you have a large frame, a weight closer to the upper range—150 pounds—may be a better target for you. Or, if you've always been overweight, whatever your frame size, then that 150-pound figure may still be a good one at which to aim. Always remember—*any* weight you can take off and keep off will be progress in the right direction.

In trying to determine your target weight, take into account what you have weighed in the past, the size of your frame, and what *you* believe is realistic. If you now weigh 175 pounds but once—perhaps ten years earlier—weighed 125 pounds, it may not be unrealistic for you to decide to aim for 125 again (provided you were at least twenty years old when you weighed 125). On the other hand, if you've never weighed less than 145 pounds since age twenty, a 30-pound weight loss is perhaps a more rational target.

If you've had a particularly hard time losing weight on other diets (or have been on numerous crash diets and now find it increasingly difficult to lose weight), the realistic thing to do is to set an initial weight-loss goal of 10 or 15 pounds. When you've lost those, set a new goal.

HOW MANY CALORIES TO MAINTAIN TARGET WEIGHT?

Once you've determined your target weight (TW), you can use the following chart to estimate the number of calories you will require each day to maintain that weight, that is, not to exceed it or go significantly under it:

Maintenance calories for men
$$725 + (31 \times TW) \text{ at age } 25$$
$$650 + (28 \times TW) \text{ at age } 45$$
$$550 + (23.5 \times TW) \text{ at age } 65$$

Maintenance calories for women
$$525 + (27 \times TW) \text{ at age } 25$$
$$475 + (24.5 \times TW) \text{ at age } 45$$
$$400 + (20.5 \times TW) \text{ at age } 65$$

Use the formula related to the age *closest* to your own age. In this formula, however, target weight must be expressed in *kilograms*. To convert the target weight you've selected to kilograms simply divide that weight in pounds by 2.2. Thus, if you are a thirty-five-year-old woman who has selected a target weight of 130 pounds, divide 130 by 2.2 and arrive at 65 kilograms. TW, for you, is 65.

(There's a twenty-year range between each category. And since you are thirty-five, you fall exactly halfway between the twenty-five- and forty-five-year-old categories. When this happens, opt for the lower category, that is, twenty-five-year-old; if you'd been thirty-six, you'd have opted for the forty-five-year-old formula.)

So, the number of calories you will need to maintain your

weight at 130 pounds (65 kilograms) is determined as follows:

$$525 + (27 \times 65)$$

Multiply 27 by 65 and you get 1755. Add 525 to 1755 to arrive at 2280, the number of calories you should consume daily to hold your weight at 130 pounds.

SOURCE OF MAINTENANCE CALORIES

Continue to use the satietizers even during the maintenance phase of your dietary program. But now *both* men and women can use the "B" satietizers. Those are the 200-calorie satietizers that are used only by men during the weight-loss phase of the program. Use one "B" satietizer before your lunch and one "B" satietizer before your dinner. The two satietizers daily will account for 400 calories. Also continue to observe the twenty-minute intrameal interval.

As before, I continue to recommend that you eat three meals a day, along with the two satietizers. Distribute the calories as you see fit among the three meals. But the more balanced the distribution the better. If you were the woman cited in the example above, who had arrived at her target weight of 130 pounds and wanted to hold it there, here's one sensible distribution you might consider:

> 480 calories breakfast
> 200 calories prelunch satietizer
> 600 calories lunch main meal
> 200 calories predinner satietizer
> 800 calories dinner main meal
> _____
> 2280 total

This distribution, of course, overlooks snacking. Snacking is discouraged during the weight-loss phase of the diet. If you return to snacking during the weight-maintenance phase, do so cautiously. *And remember to count all snack calories into your daily total.*

You can construct menu plans from the recipes included in Part Two of this book. To increase the caloric content of the portions simply divide the recipes into fewer servings. And use the calorie chart at the end of the book for further assistance in staying within your weight-maintenance allotment.

Note that the calorie chart includes the amount of fat, protein, and carbohydrate contained in different foods. Your goal, as expressed in Chapter 8, should be to get no more than 35 percent of your calories from fat. Get about 15 percent of your calories from protein and the rest from carbohydrates (at least 50 percent). Perhaps once a month or so you can run a spot-check on your daily intake to see, roughly, what the composition of your diet is. Try, as time goes along, to incorporate more and more of the low-fat/high-carbohydrate tips in Chapter 8 into your eating style. If you can eventually get your fat intake down to *below* 30 percent, more power to you. This will not only help you keep your weight down but will reduce your risk of heart disease, some cancers, and other diseases.

THE SIX FOOD GROUPS

As you select your foods, try to eat something from *each* of six food groups each day. The six groups are (1) grains and potatoes (including cereals, breads, rice, pasta, and other high-carbohydrate foods); (2) beans and legumes (almost all of us should eat more of these); (3) vegetables (try to eat fresh, steamed, or canned vegetables twice a day, at both lunch and dinner); (4) fruits (eat fresh fruit two to four times a day); (5) low-fat skim milk, yogurt made from low-fat milk, very lean meat with all visible fat removed, chicken, and fish; (6) fats (you don't really *need* to eat any foods from this group, and if you do, eat them in moderation, that is, cut back as much as you can; these foods include fatty meats, butter, salad dressings, high-fat cheeses, oils, and ice cream; replace animal fats with margarine, vegetable oil, imitation mayonnaise, and so on).

These six groups have been devised by Sonja Connor and William Connor, M.D., leading researchers on disease and diet. They are gradually supplanting the old standard "four basic food groups," which the Connors and others believe introduce too much fat into the American diet.

TIPS ON EATING AWAY FROM HOME

Eating out, whether at a restaurant or at a friend's home, has led to the demise of many a diet. The Feel Full Diet is, however, more compatible with eating out than are many weight-loss diets. For one thing, this is a mixed-nutrient, well-balanced diet. It's hard to dine out if all you're supposed to eat is pineapple. But with this diet you can eat a bit of just about everything.

First Course: Select an appetizer that complies with the standards for satietizers as outlined earlier in this book. Here are a few suggestions:

- Shrimp cocktail with regular cocktail sauce
- A few raw or steamed clams with lemon or cocktail sauce
- A small to medium bowl of chicken vegetable soup
- Clam chowder
- Smoked salmon
- Mushrooms stuffed with cheese
- Crabmeat
- Escargot
- Liver pâté

- A tossed green or Caesar salad (with 1½ tablespoons of dressing; ask for it on the side so that you don't get too much)

A Few General Reminders:

- Since you want to avoid carbohydrates during the satietizer phase of the meal, avoid eating the bread that is almost always served in restaurants ahead of the main meal.

- After finishing your satietizer, remember to observe the twenty-minute intrameal interval (you might want to tell the server to hold the main course for that long after he or she serves the satietizer).

- Alternatively, you can eat your satietizer *before* you leave for the restaurant or, as some of my patients do, *on the way to* the restaurant. Just be sure to time things so that there are at least twenty minutes between satietizer and main course. (Even if you don't get to the main course for an hour, the satietizer effect should still persist.)

Main Courses: Pay attention not only to what you are eating but also to how it is prepared.

- Avoid heavy cream sauces.
- Avoid vegetables smothered in oil, dressing, or sauces.
- Never add butter to cooked vegetables (a little margarine is okay).

Since frying foods doubles or even triples their calorie content, always try to order main courses and side dishes prepared in the following ways:

- Baked
- Smoked
- Steamed
- Broiled (do not add butter)

Dessert: If, on occasion, you still have room and, on the basis of your home experience, you believe you can afford it calorically, go ahead—indulge—but keep these suggestions in mind:

• Fresh fruit is always your best bet.

• Generally order "light" offerings.

• If you must go for a richer dessert, share it. Many people find that if they can have just one bite of a rich dessert that is enough.

• Start thinking of coffee and tea as dessert but substitute a little milk or nondairy creamer for cream. A well-brewed cup of coffee or tea can be satisfying as a final course.

These tips should come in handy particularly during the weight-maintenance phase of your diet. During the weight-loss stage, you will probably want to avoid eating out as much as possible, although if you work in an office and must eat lunches out, that can usually be done with little difficulty, provided you carry your satietizer to work with you and consume it shortly before leaving for the cafeteria or restaurant.

Finally, don't consider isolated lapses in your adherence to the diet as signs of impending failure. This diet represents a change in your way of eating and, in a very real sense, a change in your lifestyle. If you err one day you can make up for it on another. The longer you stick with the program, the easier it should become to follow.

TABLE OF FOOD COMPOSITION

The table at the back of the book (pages 217–229) provides you with the approximate composition of a large variety of different foods, listing their content of calories, protein, fat, carbohydrates, and fiber. The column at the right will be of particular use to you, telling you the total calories in some fairly typical portions of these different foods. Use this table to help you stay within the confines of your weight-maintenance program. The table will also help you avoid eating too many high-fat foods, while at the same time helping you to determine which foods are high in carbohydrates and fiber.

12

Exercise for Faster, Easier Weight Loss

(Optional *for Some*, Required *for Others*, Good *for Nearly Everybody*)

EXERCISE: WHAT ARE *YOUR* OPTIONS?

MANY PEOPLE CAN lose weight without exercising. Some others, however, absolutely *require* exercise to lose weight— and to believe otherwise is to indulge in a hopeless and possibly self-destructive delusion. Fortunately, exercise is good for nearly *everybody*, and so even those for whom it's essential to achieve lasting weight loss shouldn't regard it as punishment. The benefits of regular exercise are enormous and go far beyond weight control. Many people who exercise regularly find that they sleep better, feel better about themselves, look better, and feel more alert.

In this chapter I will spell out some of the benefits of exercise, some obvious, some not so obvious. I will help you identify what sort of person *you* are, individually—whether you are the type who can skip exercise and still lose weight (even then, you'll lose weight easier and faster if you *do* exercise) or the type who *must* exercise to lose weight. If you are one of the latter, and there are more and more of you falling into this category all the time, a careful reading of this chapter will be some of the most important and, I hope, useful reading you will ever do.

First, we'll examine the rationale for exercise in a weight-loss program. We'll examine the benefits and see who'll benefit most from exercise. Then we'll look at some specific ways of exercising that you can easily incorporate into your daily schedule without difficulty or tedium.

EXERCISING TO BURN CALORIES
(NOT AS IMPORTANT AS YOU MIGHT THINK)

If I were to ask one hundred people on the street why it's important to exercise during a weight-control program, I'm willing to bet that at least ninety-five of them would answer: "To burn calories, stupid." They'd be right—exercise *does* burn calories—but they'd be wrong in implying that this is the most important reason for exercising during dieting. Burning calories is the most obvious, direct effect of exercise.

But in reality, as many of you know, even quite a lot of exercising can burn discouragingly few calories. It can be pretty disturbing to learn that the calories you burned off while jogging a mile can be regained from eating a single milk shake or candy bar! The "return on investment" can look mighty slim to an obese person who compares "calories burned" in some fairly strenuous exercises with "calories gained" in eating some seemingly small and innocuous snacks.

So what am I saying? That exercise is a losing proposition?

Far from it. Exercise *can* and *does* burn calories, and those calories can add up, just as the snacks can. But there's a more important, less obvious reason for exercising that we're learning more about all the time. Let's see what it is.

EXERCISING TO RESET THE SET POINT

Metabolic set point is something you've perhaps heard about and perhaps also decided was too complicated to worry about. Actually, it needn't be complicated at all—and if you're serious about losing weight, you definitely need to think about it. Some have tried to present set point as a diet, almost like another fad eating program. Set point is not diet. Instead, it is a concept, describing metabolic events which, at this point, can only be manipulated through exercise. But it is a concept that works very well *in conjunction with* a well-balanced diet such as the Feel Full Diet.

The set point concept helps us to understand why so many fad diets are not only worthless but actually harmful and even fattening! It also helps us to understand why some people simply cannot lose weight using dietary measures alone. The concept is easy to grasp.

A remarkable feature of animals is their ability to maintain their "milieu interieur," or internal environment, even in the presence of harmful external factors. Even though, for example, we are exposed to ambient temperatures ranging from very cold to very hot we are able to maintain the core temperature of our bodies at 98.6°F, a temperature that promotes optimal functioning of bodily biochemical reactions. The body exerts similar controls to maintain a narrow range of blood pH, blood sugar, and blood pressure in most individuals.

The body also tries to control weight within certain predetermined, fairly narrow parameters. The set point is the weight your body strives to hold you at, *independent*, to a very large degree, of what and how much you eat. In the obese, the set point is higher than normal. Obese individuals maintain and "defend" their body weight at a high level. This is done without conscious awareness, that is, the set point is under the control of the hypothalamus, a part of the brain that regulates many functions of the body independent of conscious "will." Set point helps explain why one person on a 1200-calorie diet loses weight while another individual on the same diet does not lose and, in some instances, could even gain!

When overweight people go on diets, their decreased caloric intake and initial weight loss cause the set point to decrease their rate of energy expenditure. Their bodies become more *efficient* in holding on to weight. You cut back on calories, but the body, via the set point mechanism, still finds ways to make the most out of those calories that remain, constantly striving to keep your weight steady.

The hypothalamus, not under conscious control, doesn't know whether you have intentionally restricted food intake to lose weight or have been shipwrecked on a desert island. The hypothalamus just "assumes" you're in danger of starving and so it goes all out to maximize every last calorie you absorb. The set point might be conceived of as an ancient survival mechanism—one that helped people build up weight, some of it in the form of fat, and also hold on to it in times of food shortages.

Now that you know what an important concept set point is, don't go overboard and decide it's all-important. Set point *isn't* invincible. *Most* people, by restricting calories sufficiently, can predictably lose weight. Set point will fight you, but you can overcome it by, for example, following the Feel Full Diet. This is true for the majority of overweight individuals. Exercise, however, can help nearly *everybody* make the Feel Full Diet work even better against the set point. And, in some, exercise is *necessary* if the set point is to be made to budge.

Resetting the set point is really the most important function of exercise in a weight-loss program, though this fact has been poorly understood or not understood at all until very recently. Most fad diets ignore the whole concept of set point.

EXERCISE IS ESSENTIAL FOR MANY "YO-YO" DIETERS

"Yo-yo dieting." Ever hear of it? Maybe not. But many of you have practiced it. This is the ritual of "going on" and "going off" the latest fad diets. Many of you have probably been on several trendy diets. One woman I met had been on a *couple of dozen* over the last several years! What characterizes yo-yo dieting is losing weight, often quite a lot, and then gaining it back in a short period of time when the current diet proves no longer tolerable (usually because of overrestricted calories and/or too monotonous, unbalanced fare).

A number of health risks are now being associated with the practice of yo-yo dieting, including elevated blood pressure in some individuals. What's really awful about yo-yoing, however, is that with each new effort at dieting it becomes increasingly difficult to lose weight and increasingly easy to gain it back. Many yo-yoers actually end up weighing a little *more* at the end of each diet cycle. And where they once could perhaps lose a couple of pounds a week on a 1200-calorie-per-day diet, they now find that they can't even lose a pound a week on a dangerous 600- or 700-calorie-per-day diet. (Do you recognize yourself? Are you already a full-fledged victim of the yo-yo syndrome—or just partway there?)

Again, these unfortunate individuals are still in the minority, but more and more of them are coming to my attention and to that of other physicians all the time. And, once again, the set point mechanism is involved—only here it is truly running amok because of the dietary abuse to which it has repeatedly been subjected.

Is all lost? Is the damage irreversible? No one knows if *all* of the damage can be reversed, but it is evident that much of it can be—if the individual turns to and sticks with a *prudent, balanced* diet *combined with an equally prudent program of exercise.* Once you're really on the yo-yo treadmill, this combination is probably the *only* way out of your serious dilemma.

And exercise, as I've said several times, can help *everybody* combat the effects of the well-intentioned but counterproductive set point. There is growing and quite convincing evidence that, apart from burning calories, there may be a residual effect of exercise, one that increases the basal metabolic rate for up to forty-eight hours after the exercise is over. Now that is a truly great "return on investment." By exercising thirty to sixty minutes just three to five times per week, you might achieve an effect that makes it more difficult for your body to hold on to excess calories even while you sleep.

OTHER ADVANTAGES OF EXERCISE

We're talking here about the advantages of exercise *while trying to lose weight.* Obviously, there are general advantages of exercise; improving the quality of heart/lung function is a major one. Recently, an ambitious study led by researchers at the Harvard School of Public Health demonstrated that regular exercise *markedly* reduces the risks of breast cancer and cancers of the reproductive system in women. Even fairly moderate exercise was found to exert a protective influence. There is reason to believe that obese women are at even greater risk than other women of developing these cancers, indicating a pressing need for exercise among overweight women. Obesity is also a significant risk factor related to various cancers and especially cardiovascular disease in men.

But, in addition to all this, and to the effects of exercise on calories and the set point, there are other benefits to be derived from increased physical activity during weight loss. Simple dieting, without exercise, tends to cut into lean body mass more than does a combination of dieting and exercise. The combination of exercise with dieting encourages the body to burn fat while retaining and building muscle.

In addition, moderate exercise can reduce rather than stimulate the appetite. So don't be too concerned that walking for an hour burns only about 325 calories. You will benefit from exercise in so many ways that it is well worth the walk.

EXERCISE: FIRST ASSUME THE RIGHT ATTITUDE

Given the way so many of us live, it's not always easy to get into an exercise frame of mind. In our high-tech society brilliant minds are continually at work dreaming up new inventions to help us avoid physical exertion. We've come a long way from the era of washing clothes on scrub boards and walking five miles (barefoot) to school. Now we have elevators, garage door openers, electric can openers, central vacuuming systems, and, of course, the ever-present automobile.

How many times have you waited irritating minutes for the elevator to go a couple of flights when the nearby stairs stood waiting and empty? How many times have you navigated through the maze of a shopping mall parking lot for ten or twenty minutes to find a space close to the door so you wouldn't have to walk a block? Even those who make exercising a part of their daily lives fall prey to these lazy habits. There are those of us who will regularly play five sets of tennis but drive the car three blocks to the courts.

Incorporating exercise into one's life can be simple. Although I will outline some formal exercise options, I will also make some suggestions for exercising without really trying. The best way to start is to welcome instead of to avoid walking that block or those three blocks, taking the stairs, and so forth. Dreaded chores—such as weeding the garden—can become exercise opportunities. Wallpapering, mowing lawns, mopping floors, painting, raking leaves, walking instead of driving to the store—they all add up.

Such "casual" exercises are to be encouraged along with a more formal exercise routine practiced three to five times per week. Before you start any regular exercise program you should consult your physician. This is especially important if you are more than 20 percent above your ideal body weight (see the chapter on weight maintenance to determine your ideal weight). It is also important if you are a male over thirty with a family history of heart disease, if you are over forty, or if you have a preexisting medical problem. None of these factors will necessarily rule out an exercise program and, in fact, may make one even more important—but that's for your doctor to help you decide on an individual basis.

TIPS ON STARTING AN EXERCISE PROGRAM

1. *Start slowly.* If you are an armchair athlete now, you will not become an Olympic champion in a week. Although the program should be stimulating, you should not push too hard.

Below is a chart listing the average *maximum* pulse rate that should be achieved by strenuous exercise. This chart is based on an individual with a resting pulse rate of 70 beats per minute. If your resting pulse rate is lower than 70 BPM, these numbers would be slightly lower. Likewise, if your resting pulse rate is higher than 70 BPM these figures would be elevated slightly.

Resting Pulse = 70 BPM

AGE	25	35	45	55	65
AVERAGE MAXIMUM BPM	157	150	143	136	129

If you find that exercising elevates your pulse beyond the maximum BPM, you should *reduce* your exercise load. By gradually building up your program, you will be able to increase your workout without raising your heart rate above the maximum BPM.

It is advisable to know your pulse rate during strenuous exercise. If you aren't sure how to take your pulse, ask your physician for instruction.

2. *Set aside specific times* for a workout. Although your workout may vary from day to day, it is wise to have a schedule for exercising. This will help eliminate the old excuse, "I didn't have time." If you plan for regular exercise there will always be time.

3. *Don't plan strenuous exercise* immediately after a meal. A workout on a full stomach can cause cramps, nausea, and heartburn. Therefore, it is wise to wait at least one hour after eating before commencing exercise. Many people find they are not very hungry following strenuous exercise, so you may want to schedule your workout for times you normally like to snack.

This tip does not rule out the possibility of light-to-moderate exercise after the satietizer portion of your meal. A twenty-minute walk can be a productive way to spend the waiting period between the satietizer and main course during an office lunch hour.

4. *Set goals.* After you have maintained an exercise program you will notice improvement in your performance. Don't take the easy way out by remaining at the beginner's level. Set realistic goals that will allow you to increase your exercise program, thereby lowering your set point, burning extra calories, and making you thinner!

5. *Monitor your progress.* There is nothing more rewarding than watching your performance increase as you watch your weight decrease! Keep a chart of your goals and achievements. If you exercise in different ways, keep a separate entry for each activity.

6. *Don't get discouraged* if your progress slows. Just as with dieting, you may notice rapid improvement followed by slower progress. Don't give up! The point of exercising is just that: to exercise. You are not training to be a world-class athlete but are exercising to lose weight and improve your health.

7. *Wear appropriate clothing.* Loose-fitting, comfortable clothes will aid you in your exercising endeavor. Tight jeans or flapping dresses will only hamper your progress and make you uncomfortable. You may even want to buy a new outfit that is appropriate for your workout. If you look good, you'll feel good and you'll be ready to work out.

8. *Vary your exercise routine.* Unless you find an exercise you like to do day after day that doesn't get monotonous, engage in different exercise activities to avoid boredom. You might decide to swim one day a week, walk two days, play tennis on another day, and so forth. Of course, there's nothing *wrong* with walking five days a week, and I encourage you to do so if you enjoy it. The point is that you don't *have* to do the same exercise each day.

9. *Consider finding an exercise partner* or joining an exercise group. Having a jogging or walking partner, for example, can help keep you motivated. If your enthusiasm for exercise reaches a low ebb, your partner can prod you into action; you can do the same for him or her. Also, it makes the time pass more quickly to have someone along to talk to on a walk. There are many exercise groups in most communities —swimming clubs, walking and hiking clubs, dance aerobics classes, and so on. These, too, can help keep motivation at a peak. On the other hand, you may enjoy solo exercising, and that's fine, too. Some people find exercising alone gives them the privacy to clear their minds, work out problems, even plan weekly menus!

SPECIFIC EXERCISE OPTIONS

Let's look now at some specific exercises you may want to consider.

Walking: Walking is one of the best and most ignored exercises for either a beginning or a more advanced workout. Walking is great because it allows us to exercise while we enjoy the scenery we miss as we zoom by in our cars. The only equipment necessary is a pair of comfortable shoes. I recommend running shoes, which are available in a wide range of styles and prices. Running shoes offer the support and cushioning ideal for a brisk walk. Your walking speed should be brisk enough to elevate your pulse rate—but not so brisk that it pushes your pulse up beyond your maximum BPM discussed earlier in this chapter. Vary your route from time to time to prevent boredom. Gradually increase your pace and/or the distance you cover. And remember: walking a mile at a good pace burns nearly the same number of calories as jogging a mile! And walking is easier on the joints.

Jogging: Jogging, like walking, requires little equipment and is great exercise. Once again, wear running shoes for comfort and support. Jogging, in addition to burning calories, will increase the performance of your cardiovascular system. If you are a beginner, start jogging by incorporating it into your walking program. Many people increase their jogging distances by plotting a walk/jog course: walk a portion of the course, then jog a portion, alternating walking and jogging until the course is completed. Increase the jogging segment while decreasing the walking until the entire course can be run. This strategy can be employed to increase your distances as well. Some experts feel that jogging on a track or similar soft surface is better than jogging on a hard streetlike surface. You may find grassy surfaces along the road to be a comfortable course.

Jumping Rope: Jumping rope is no longer just a child's game! It is a great way to exercise, and it can be done indoors or outside. Good, supportive athletic shoes and a jump rope are all the equipment you need. Start out slowly and increase your exercise by increasing the time you jump. You will find it more comfortable to jump on grassy surfaces or a padded rug. For an added dimension to your workout, try jumping to music. Select music with a tempo compatible with your jumping speed. You can change tunes as you increase your workout speed and duration. Start slowly. Jumping rope can be strenuous.

Exercise Routines (*Calisthenics*): Although an exercise routine often drums up images of TV exercise shows at 5 A.M., the exercise routine can be fun if it is tailored to your individual needs. The most effective routines are diverse enough to cover all parts of the body. They should begin with a warm-up, go on to exercise the arms, waist, legs/hips, and buttocks, and end with a cool-down. It is also helpful to include an aerobic or dance segment in the routine. Music can often make the difference between a dull routine and an invigorating one. Keep in mind that the tempo of the music must coordinate with the routine.

Skiing: Both downhill and cross-country skiing are fun winter sports that burn calories. Both are great for leg conditioning, and cross-country skiing is especially good for your cardiovascular system. Although downhill skiing requires a certain level of expertise, cross-country can be learned rapidly and does not require the hills of a ski resort. In fact, it is the perfect exercise for anyone in a snowy climate because it allows you to enjoy the scenery as well as to benefit from the exercise.

Tennis: Singles tennis can be an enjoyable and effective way to exercise, but remember, you have to run around the court to get benefit from the sport! Just waiting for the ball to come to you defeats the opportunity for a workout and will probably cost you the game. Doubles tennis is a less effective way to work out but may be good for the beginner. There is less running involved and therefore the workout benefits are reduced.

Cycling: With cycling, either on a stationary or mobile bicycle, the legs and cardiovascular system get a real workout. Stationary bikes offer many of the benefits of a regular bike but also have the added convenience of being "weatherproof." Some sophisticated bikes can be programmed to "go up and down hills," calculate calorie consumption, and indicate the time and distance traveled. Remember that exercising on a stationary bike allows you the freedom to read or watch TV while you work out.

Swimming: Swimming is one of the best exercises there is. It exercises the whole body but puts little stress on the joints. You can swim straight laps or circle laps (permitted at some pools) or do your own thing if you have access to your own pool or are near an ocean, lake, or swimmable river. Always observe water-safety rules.

Rowing Machines: Rowing machines provide an excellent workout for the arms, abdomen, legs, and cardiovascular system. In addition, they provide a workout in a relatively short period of time—fifteen to thirty minutes. There are several variations of rowing machines on the market, but the best ones feature sliding seats and dual rowing arms. Some models will even calculate the number of calories you are burning as you stroke.

HOW MUCH TO EXERCISE

Exercise *regularly*. Five times a week is best but three exercise sessions will be adequate. If you engage in brisk stationary cycling or rowing fifteen or twenty minutes per exercise session, three times a week may be adequate. Walking and jogging will be more productive if they are in the half-hour to hour range each session.

Although the consumption of calories is only one of the benefits derived from exercise, this factor does provide a means of comparing different exercises. The table below shows you the number of calories burned in one hour spent engaged in different exercises. These are "ballpark" estimates because each individual will differ a little. Note that these figures are for individuals weighing 150 to 200 pounds. You can make educated guesses as to your own caloric expenditures by extrapolating from these figures based on your own weight.

	CALORIES BURNED/HOUR	
	150-pound	*200-pound*
Activity	*person*	*person*
Aerobic dancing	685	930
Cycling (9 mph)	400	540
Golf	340	360
Running (11.5 min/mile)	550	732
Swimming freestyle	630	850
Tennis (singles)	445	600
Walking	325	430

Keep in mind that the exercises listed above are just a few of the many available to you. And to keep your motivation high, remember that exercise benefits you in many ways—by burning calories, lowering set point, reducing appetite, conditioning muscles, lessening the risk of a variety of diseases, and so on.

And, finally, remember that just as the Feel Full Diet is more a lifestyle change than a momentary aberration in diet, so should your exercise program become a permanent part of your life. The longer you stick with your new eating and exercising habits, the easier they will become and the better you'll look and feel.

II

The Feel Full Meal
Plan and Recipes

Recipes and Menus by
Gloria Kaufer Greene

CONTENTS

CHAPTER 15 — MAIN DISHES — MEAT

CHAPTER 16—MAIN DISHES—POULTRY

CHAPTER 17—MAIN DISHES—FISH AND SHELLFISH

CHAPTER 18 — MAIN DISHES— VEGETARIAN

CHAPTER 19 — SIDE DISHES AND QUICK BREADS

CHAPTER 20 — BREAKFAST DISHES

CHAPTER 21 — DESSERTS

13

The Fourteen-Day
Feel Full Menu Plan

THE FOLLOWING FOURTEEN-DAY menu plan will introduce you to the delicious variety of foods possible within the
guidelines of the Feel Full Diet. Recipes for most of these dishes
are included in the next several chapters. An asterisk (*) indicates that the recipe is included in this book. These sample
menus deliver approximately 1200 calories per day—the caloric intake prescribed for women under the "standard" program. Each of the satietizers used in these menus is valued at
150 calories, but they can be increased to 200 calories to provide the "standard" 1300 calories for men. Each of the satietizer recipes (provided in the next chapter) specifies both 150-
and 200-calorie portions. The numbers that follow each main
course, side dish, or dessert entry are the calories per serving.

You may choose to follow these menus exactly—or you may
decide to make substitutions (one item for another with equal
calories). There may actually be more variety here than you

want—at least in the beginning. Some of my patients pick out menus for two, three, or four of the fourteen days and concentrate on those for a week or two before moving on to "new days." That's perfectly all right because each sample day provides for well-balanced fare.

These menu plans are meant to provide inspiration and example. From the recipes provided in subsequent chapters, you can begin putting together your own daily plans—right from the start, if you so desire. Just remember to follow the general guidelines detailed in Part One of this book and particularly those dealt with in the chapters on the satietizers and main courses.

I think, though, that when you look at these menus you'll want to try most, if not all, of these combinations. Who says dieting has to be boring? It's breakfast. Pass me my Wake-Up Banana Split!

Note: Coffee, tea, seltzer, or water may be consumed with any breakfast.

DAY 1

	calories
Breakfast	
*Fluffy Whole Wheat Buttermilk Pancakes	165
½ large navel orange or 1 fresh peach	40
Lunch	
*Yellow Squash Bisque (satietizer)	150
*Gingered Chicken Salad in Pita Bread	280
1 cup skim milk	90

calories

Dinner

* Whole Stuffed Artichoke (satietizer)	150
* Swiss Steak Dinner with Vegetables	270
* Frozen Banana Fudgies	55
	1200

Day 2

Breakfast

* Wake-Up Banana Split	205

Lunch

* Nutty Popcorn Mix (satietizer)	150
* Hearty New England–Style Fish Chowder	225
4 whole wheat melba toasts	60
Green salad with 1 tablespoon reduced-calorie dressing	35

Dinner

* Cheesy Crab Dip (satietizer)	150
* Zucchini Lasagne	280
1 cup skim milk	90
	1195

DAY 3

calories

Breakfast

1 ounce (⅓ cup) granola	125
1 cup skim milk	90

Lunch

*Herbed Deviled Eggs (satietizer)	150
*Pasta with Sherried Shrimp	230
*Sesame Broccoli with Mock Hollandaise Sauce	55

Dinner

*Savory Ricotta Snacks (satietizer)	150
*Turkey with Wine and Mushrooms	180
*Lemony New Potatoes	95
⅔ cup cooked carrots	30
*Micro-Baked Stuffed Apple	95
	1200

DAY 4

Breakfast

*Fresh Fruit with Orange–Poppy-Seed Dressing	180

	calories
Lunch	
*Quick Beef and Vegetable Soup (satietizer)	150
*Broiled Herbed Chicken Breasts	155
*Red Cabbage and Apples	60
*Whole Wheat Irish Soda Bread with	
1 teaspoon reduced-calorie margarine	115
Dinner	
*Cottage Sundae (satietizer)	150
*Poached Turbot with Mirepoix Sauce	160
6 to 8 brussels sprouts, boiled or steamed	35
1 medium-sized (about 6 ounces) baked	
potato	110
*Pineapple Sherbet	75
	1190

DAY 5

Breakfast	
1 large shredded wheat biscuit	85
1 cup skim milk	90
2 apricot halves in light syrup	35

Lunch	
*Sherried Chicken Liver Paté (satietizer)	150
*Molded Salmon-Cucumber Salad	225

	calories
*Raisin-Bran Muffin with 1 teaspoon reduced-calorie margarine	90
¾ cup fresh strawberries	35

Dinner

*Cottage Dip with Crudités (satietizer)	150
*Sweet-and-Sour Ground Beef and Cabbage	245
½ cup cooked egg noodles	100
	1205

DAY 6

Breakfast

*Dutch Apple Pancake	210

Lunch

*Tuna in a Tomato "Flower" (satietizer)	150
*Hearty Lentil Soup/Stew	265
2 triple rye crisp crackers	50

Dinner

*Ricotta "Cheesecakes" (satietizer)	150
*Chicken Cacciatore (with spaghetti)	290

calories

*Easy Ratatouille	65
½ cup grapes	30
	1210

DAY 7

Breakfast

1 cup cooked oatmeal	130
½ cup skim milk	45
1 dried fig	40

Lunch

*Spring Salad (satietizer)	150
*Baked Potatoes with Tuna Florentine	
Topping	285
2 medium-sized raw carrots, cut into sticks	60

Dinner

*Egg Drop Soup (satietizer)	150
*Oriental Beef and Broccoli (with rice)	265
*Strawberries and "Cream"	75
	1195

DAY 8

	calories
Breakfast	
*Cottage Cheese Pancakes	190
Lunch	
*Seafarer's Tomato Soup (satietizer)	150
*Broccoli Frittata	235
Green salad with 1 tablespoon reduced-calorie dressing	35
1 cup skim milk	90
Dinner	
*In-a-Minute Miniature Pizza (satietizer)	150
*Garden Mini Meat Loaves	220
½ cup mashed potatoes with 1 teaspoon reduced-calorie margarine	95
*Braised Parmesan Celery	30
	1195

DAY 9

Breakfast	
*Mock Cheese Danish	195
Lunch	
*Sassy Sardine-Stuffed Celery (satietizer)	150
*Turkey-Sprout Waldorf Salad	215

	calories
*Raisin-Bran Muffin with 1 teaspoon reduced-calorie margarine	90
1 cup skim milk	90

Dinner

*Herbed Neufchâtel Cheese (satietizer)	150
*Creole-Style Fish Dinner (with rice)	250
*Meringue Pears Melba	55
	1195

DAY 10

Breakfast

*French Toast with Orange-Raisin Sauce	215
½ cup skim milk	45

Lunch

*Whole Wheat Sesame Crackers (satietizer)	150
*Easy Pumpkin Soup	65
*Zucchini Halves Stuffed with Tuna	230
1 small apple cut into wedges and sprinkled with ground cinnamon	60

Dinner

*Rumaki (satietizer)	150
*Oven-Barbecued Chicken	170
*Country Coleslaw	55
*Easiest-Ever Raspberry Sherbet	50
	1190

DAY 11

	calories
Breakfast	
½ grapefruit, peeled and cut into chunks	40
* 1 Raisin-Bran Muffin	75
1 cup skim milk	90
Lunch	
*Viennese Cheese Dumplings (satietizer)	150
*Crab and Rice Salad	240
*Sesame Broccoli with Mock Hollandaise Sauce	55
Dinner	
*Peanut Soup (satietizer)	150
*Marinated Flank Steak with Vegetable Kebabs	260
½ cup hot cooked rice	90
*"Ice-Cream" Banana Pop	50
	1200

DAY 12

Breakfast	
*Fruity Cooked Cream of Wheat	215
Lunch	
*Peanut Butter Crackles (satietizer)	150
*Baked Potatoes with Dilled Dairy Topping	270

	calories
1 small fresh pear or 2 small canned pear halves in juice	60

Dinner

*Mushroom-Walnut Spread (satietizer)	150
*Sweet-and-Sour Cabbage Soup	55
*Sole and Asparagus Bundles	160
*Easy Ratatouille	65
*Molded Prune Whip	70
	1195

DAY 13

Breakfast

*Strawberry and Cheese Crêpes	200

Lunch

*Peanut Butter–Honey Balls (satietizer)	150
*Chinese-Style Chicken and Vegetables (with rice)	280
1 large plum or peach	45

Dinner

*Nachos with Cheese (satietizer)	150
*Chili con Carne	270
*Corn Muffin with 1 teaspoon reduced-calorie margarine	105
	1200

DAY 14

	calories
Breakfast	
1 cup low-fat vanilla, lemon, or coffee yogurt	200

Lunch

* Chinese-Style Hot-and-Sour Soup (satietizer)	150
* Seafood Egg Fou Yong (with rice)	260
1 tablespoon raisins	25

Dinner

* Brie with Almonds (satietizer)	150
* Turkey Normandy	220
½ cup hot, cooked egg noodles	100
10 medium-sized cooked fresh asparagus spears	25
* Piña Colada Chiffon Squares	70
	1200

14

Satietizers

IN THE RECIPES in this chapter, "A" servings are 150 calories and are for women; "B" servings are 200 calories and are for men. Amounts in parentheses are for "B" servings.

All recipes should be divided into *equal* servings for calorie counts to be correct.

YELLOW SQUASH BISQUE

3 tablespoons reduced-calorie margarine
1 large onion, finely chopped
4 medium-sized yellow squash [about 1⅓ pounds], cubed
1⅓ cups water
1 chicken or vegetable bouillon cube or envelope of powder
½ teaspoon dried basil leaves
⅛ teaspoon dried thyme leaves
Pinch of ground black pepper (or to taste)
⅔ cup instant nonfat dry milk powder
⅓ cup cool water

119

TO SERVE:

4 tablespoons commercial sour cream
Fresh or dried chopped chives

In a large saucepan, melt the margarine over medium-high heat; add the onion and cook, stirring constantly, until it is tender but not browned. Add the squash and continue cooking, stirring constantly, for 2 minutes. Add the 1⅓ cups water, bouillon cube or powder, herbs, and pepper. Cover the saucepan, reduce the heat, and simmer for about 15 minutes or until the squash is tender. Remove from the heat and let cool to lukewarm. Purée the soup, in batches, in a blender or food processor. Return to the saucepan.

In a large cup, mix the milk powder into the ⅓ cup cool water until completely dissolved; then stir it into the soup. Cook the soup, stirring, over medium heat until it is heated through. Ladle into bowls and top each serving with 1 table-spoon (1⅓ tablespoons) sour cream. Sprinkle chives on the sour cream.

Makes 4 "A" (3 "B") satietizer servings.

EGG DROP SOUP

1 cup canned or homemade chicken broth (not bouillon), sea-
   soned to taste
1½ teaspoons cornstarch
1 tablespoon water
1 large egg, lightly beaten
1 scallion, including green top, thinly sliced on the diagonal
1½ tablespoons (3 tablespoons) chow mein noodles

Put the broth in a small saucepan and bring to a boil over medium-high heat. Combine the cornstarch and water and add, stirring, to the broth. Stir until the broth clears and thickens slightly. Slowly pour the beaten egg into the broth while stirring constantly. Continue to cook and stir the soup briefly until the egg forms threads. Stir in the scallion. Serve hot with the noodles.

Makes 1 "A" (1 "B") satietizer serving.

FRESH GREEN PEA SOUP

2 tablespoons reduced-calorie margarine
1 small onion, finely chopped
¾ cup chicken or vegetable bouillon made from cubes or
  powder
3 cups loose-pack frozen green peas
¼ teaspoon dried marjoram leaves
¼ teaspoon dried thyme leaves
⅛ teaspoon salt
Pinch of ground black or white pepper
1½ cups skim milk
2 teaspoons flour

In a large saucepan, melt the margarine over medium-high heat; add the onion and cook until it is tender but not browned. Add the bouillon, peas, herbs, salt, and pepper and bring the mixture to a boil. Remove from the heat and stir in ¼ cup of the milk. Purée the pea mixture in a blender or food processor (in batches, if necessary) until it is very smooth. If the mixture is too thick to purée easily, add a little more milk. Pour the purée back into the saucepan. Mix the flour with the remaining milk until no lumps remain. Add the flour-milk mixture to the puréed peas and cook the soup, stirring, until it comes to a boil. Reduce the heat and simmer for 2 minutes.

Makes 4 "A" (3 "B") satietizer servings.

PEANUT SOUP

1 small onion, finely chopped
1 small potato, peeled and diced
1 medium-sized tomato, peeled, seeded, and diced
2 tablespoons uncooked white rice
2 cups chicken or vegetable bouillon made from cubes or
    powder
¼ cup smooth or crunchy peanut butter
3 tablespoons instant nonfat dry milk powder
¼ cup water
⅛ teaspoon ground black pepper
Pinch of salt

In a medium-sized saucepan, combine the onion, potato, to-mato, rice, and bouillon. Bring to a boil over high heat, reduce the heat, and simmer, covered, for about 20 minutes or until the potato and rice are just tender. In a small bowl, combine the peanut butter, milk powder, and water and mix until smooth. Stir into the soup, along with the pepper and salt. Cook, stirring occasionally, for about 5 minutes longer. Purée half the contents of the saucepan in a blender or food processor. Return the purée to the saucepan and mix well. Continue cooking until heated through.

Makes 4 "A" (3 "B") satietizer servings.

QUICK BEEF AND VEGETABLE SOUP

8 ounces extra-lean ground beef
1 [16-ounce] can plain tomato sauce
2 cups beef bouillon made from cubes or powder
1½ cups cut-up fresh or frozen mixed vegetables, including
    broccoli, cauliflower, green beans, and/or carrots
1 celery stalk, thinly sliced
3 tablespoons chopped fresh parsley leaves
1 teaspoon dried basil leaves
1 teaspoon dried marjoram leaves
⅛ teaspoon ground black pepper

In a large saucepan, brown the beef over medium-high heat while breaking it up with a spoon. Add the remaining ingredients and bring to a boil. Reduce the heat and simmer for 8 to 10 minutes or until the vegetables are tender but not mushy.

Makes 4 "A" (3 "B") satietizer servings.

SEAFARER'S TOMATO SOUP

3 tablespoons reduced-calorie margarine
1 small onion, finely chopped
2 celery stalks, thinly sliced
1½ tablespoons all-purpose flour
1 [24-ounce] can OR 2 [12-ounce] cans vegetable-tomato juice
2 scallions, including green tops, thinly sliced
½ teaspoon dried basil leaves
¼ teaspoon dried thyme leaves
1 [5-ounce] package frozen tiny cooked shrimp OR 1 [4½-
    ounce] can shrimp, rinsed and drained

TO SERVE:

28 (27) small oyster crackers

In a medium-sized saucepan, melt the margarine over medium-high heat; then sauté the onion and celery until tender. Add the flour and stir until it is well mixed with the vegetables. Slowly add the juice, stirring constantly to avoid lumps. Add the scallions, basil, and thyme and continue cooking, stirring often, until the soup comes to a boil and thickens slightly. Reduce the heat and simmer 1 minute. Add the shrimp. Continue simmering the soup, stirring, for 1 to 2 minutes or until the shrimp is just heated through. Float 7 (9) oyster crackers on each serving of soup.

Makes 4 "A" (3 "B") satietizer servings.

CHINESE-STYLE HOT-AND-SOUR SOUP

5 ounces boneless lean pork or beef, trimmed of all surface fat,
    thinly sliced, and cut into narrow julienne strips
3 cups canned chicken broth (not bouillon)
1 tablespoon soy sauce
1 cup sliced fresh mushrooms OR 1 [3- to 4-ounce] can mush-
    rooms, drained
1 [8-ounce] can sliced bamboo shoots, drained and rinsed
1½ tablespoons white vinegar
⅛ to ¼ teaspoon ground black or white pepper
1½ tablespoons cornstarch
2 tablespoons cold water
1 large egg, lightly beaten
1 scallion, including green top, thinly sliced on the diagonal

Coat a medium-sized saucepan with nonstick cooking spray and heat over medium-high heat; add the pork or beef and cook, stirring constantly, until just cooked through. Add the broth, soy sauce, mushrooms, and bamboo shoots and bring to a boil. Reduce heat and simmer for 2 to 3 minutes or until the mushrooms are cooked. Add the vinegar and pepper. Mix the cornstarch and water and add to the soup. Cook, stirring, until the soup thickens slightly, then slowly pour in the egg while stirring constantly. Cook until the egg forms threads. Sprinkle the scallion on top and serve.

Makes 4 "A" (3 "B") satietizer servings.

COTTAGE DIP WITH CRUDITÉS

1 cup 1% fat cottage cheese
1 cup low-fat plain yogurt
¼ cup reduced-calorie mayonnaise
¼ cup finely chopped scallions, including green tops
2 tablespoons finely chopped fresh parsley leaves
1 teaspoon dried dill leaves
¼ teaspoon dried basil leaves
¼ teaspoon powdered mustard
Salt and black pepper to taste

TO SERVE:
Raw vegetables such as celery stalks, sliced cucumber or raw zucchini, raw mushrooms, sliced green pepper, broccoli or cauliflower florets, or carrot sticks

Put the cottage cheese in a medium-sized bowl and mash any large curds with a fork. Stir in the remaining ingredients and chill, covered, several hours to let the flavors blend. May be refrigerated up to three days.) Serve with raw vegetables (crudités).

Makes 4 "A" (3 "B") satietizer servings.

HERBED DEVILED EGGS

3 hard-boiled eggs, shelled
3 tablespoons reduced-calorie mayonnaise
½ teaspoon dried tarragon or thyme leaves (or other herb to
 taste)
½ teaspoon white or wine vinegar
¼ teaspoon powdered mustard
Pinch of paprika
Pinch of black pepper
2 tablespoons finely chopped fresh parsley leaves

Cut each egg in half lengthwise and carefully remove the yolks. Put the yolk pieces in a bowl and mash with a fork. Stir in the mayonnaise, herbs, vinegar, mustard, paprika, and pepper. Spoon the mixture into the egg-white halves, heaping it in the center. Sprinkle the parsley on top. 1 "A" serving = 2 halves. (1 "B" serving = 3 halves.)

Makes 3 "A" (2 "B") satietizer servings.

PEANUT BUTTER—HONEY BALLS

⅓ cup instant nonfat dry milk powder
4½ tablespoons smooth or crunchy peanut butter
1½ tablespoons honey
1½ tablespoons unsweetened cocoa OR nonfat dry milk
 powder

In a medium-sized bowl, combine the ⅓ cup milk powder, peanut butter, and honey and mix well to form a pliable dough that is neither crumbly nor sticky. If the mixture is very dry, add water, drop by drop, until it is the right consistency. If it is too sticky, add a few pinches of milk powder. Form the mixture into

12 equal balls (or roll it into a 12-inch log and cut into 1-inch slices). Coat the balls (or slices) with the cocoa or additional milk powder. If desired, the balls (or slices) may be stored in an airtight container in the refrigerator for 2 weeks or longer. 1 "A" serving = 3 balls (1 "B" serving = 4 balls).

Makes 4 "A" (3 "B") satietizer servings.

WHOLE WHEAT SESAME CRACKERS

½ cup whole wheat flour
2 tablespoons stick butter or margarine (NOT reduced-calorie)
2 tablespoons sesame seeds OR hulled, unsalted sunflower seeds
⅛ teaspoon salt
½ cup 1% fat cottage cheese

Put the flour, butter, sesame (or sunflower) seeds, and salt into a food processor fitted with the steel blade and pulse-process until the mixture looks like fine crumbs. Transfer to a small bowl. Add the cottage cheese to the food processor and process until smooth. Return the flour mixture and process until a ball forms.

Coat a large, flat cookie sheet (or the bottom of an inverted pan) well with nonstick cooking spray. Roll out the dough very thinly on the cookie sheet or pan bottom to an approximate 13-by 10-inch rectangle. Be careful not to make the edges thinner than the center. Prick the dough all over with a fork. Use a pastry wheel, pizza cutter, or sharp knife to cut the rectangle crosswise into 4 equal strips and then lengthwise into 3 equal strips to make 12 equal rectangles. Next, cut each rectangle equally into fourths, for a total of 48 crackers.

Bake the crackers in a 325°F oven for about 20 minutes or

until they are browned and crisp. If those on the edges get done first, remove them and continue baking the remainder. Cool the crackers in one layer on a wire rack. 1 "A" serving = 12 small crackers. (1 "B" serving = 16 small crackers.)

Makes 4 "A" (3 "B") satietizer servings.

P.B.J. CRACKERS

1 tablespoon (1 tablespoon + 1 teaspoon) peanut butter
4 (6) Whole Wheat Sesame Crackers (see page 127) OR 3 (4)
    Ritz crackers (or similar small crackers)
1 teaspoon (1½ teaspoons) reduced-calorie (low-sugar) jam or
    preserves

Spread the peanut butter on the crackers, dividing it evenly. Top with a dab of the jam.

Makes 1 "A" (1 "B") satietizer serving.

COTTAGE SUNDAE

½ cup (⅔ cup) 1% fat cottage cheese
3 tablespoons (¼ cup) unsweetened applesauce
1 tablespoon chopped walnuts
Pinch of ground cinnamon (optional)

Use a large ice cream scoop (or a spoon) to form the cottage cheese into a mound in a dessert dish. Spoon the applesauce on top and sprinkle with the walnuts and cinnamon (if desired).

Makes 1 "A" (1 "B") satietizer serving.

LACY CHEESE WAFERS

1½ ounces (2 ounces) cheddar, longhorn, or Monterey jack cheese, cut into 3 (4) slices

Line a baking sheet with foil; then coat the foil with nonstick cooking spray. Place the cheese slices 3 inches apart on the foil. Bake in a preheated 350°F oven for 5 to 8 minutes or until the cheese is bubbly and lightly browned. Lift the foil from the baking sheet and set on the countertop for about 1 minute so the wafers can firm up slightly. Gently peel the wafers off the foil and place them on paper towels to absorb excess fat. The wafers crisp more as they cool. (They may be made in larger quantities and stored in an airtight container for 2 to 3 days.)

Makes 1 "A" (1 "B") satietizer serving.

SASSY SARDINE-STUFFED CELERY

1 [3¾-ounce] can sardines in mustard sauce, drained
2 hard-boiled eggs, coarsely chopped
2 tablespoons finely chopped fresh parsley leaves
3 tablespoons reduced-calorie mayonnaise
2 teaspoons tarragon vinegar (or wine vinegar) (or to taste)
½ teaspoon prepared mustard, preferably brown (or to taste)
¼ teaspoon onion powder
Ground black pepper to taste

TO SERVE:
Celery sticks (as many as desired)

In a medium-sized bowl, combine the spread ingredients, mashing thoroughly with a fork. For a smoother spread, purée the mixture in a food processor or food mill. Spoon the spread into celery sticks. Refrigerate in an airtight container for up to 4 days.

Makes 4 "A" (3 "B") satietizer servings.

HERBED CHEESE OMELET SLICES

1 large egg
1 teaspoon water
½ teaspoon finely chopped fresh parsley leaves
¼ teaspoon dried thyme leaves
¼ teaspoon dried basil leaves
Dash of hot red pepper sauce (or a pinch of ground black pepper)
Pinch of salt
¾ ounce (1¼ ounces) American cheese (or similar process cheese), thinly sliced or grated

With a fork, beat the egg and water together until they are light and very well mixed. Beat in the herbs, hot pepper sauce, and salt. Preheat a 7- to 8-inch-diameter skillet over medium-high heat, then coat it with nonstick vegetable spray. Add the egg mixture and tilt the pan so that the egg covers the bottom. Cook 30 seconds to 1 minute or until the egg is almost dry on top. Reduce the heat if the bottom is browning too fast. Put the cheese on top of the egg, cover the skillet, and reduce the heat to low. Continue cooking about 30 seconds or until the cheese is melted. Transfer the omelet to a plate, cheese side up, and roll it up tightly. Let it cool for a few seconds to hold its shape, then slice on the diagonal into 4 pieces.

Makes 1 "A" (1 "B") satietizer serving.

CHEESY CRAB DIP

1 [6½-ounce] can crabmeat, drained
½ cup 1% fat cottage cheese
¼ cup commercial sour cream
2 tablespoons reduced-calorie mayonnaise
1 teaspoon prepared mustard
1 teaspoon lemon juice
Dash of Worcestershire sauce
Dash of hot red pepper sauce
Pinch of paprika

TO SERVE:
8 (9) whole wheat melba toasts

Process the dip ingredients in a food processor fitted with a steel blade or beat them together with an electric mixer until well combined. For each serving, use one-fourth (one-third) of the dip with 2 (3) melba toasts. Refrigerate extra dip in a covered container for up to 4 days.

Makes 4 "A" (3 "B") satietizer servings.

BRIE WITH ALMONDS

1¼ ounces (1½ ounces) brie or camembert cheese
4 (6) plain soda crackers or matzo crackers
1 teaspoon sliced almonds

Divide the cheese into 4 (6) small pieces and put one piece on each cracker. Sprinkle the almonds over the cheese. Heat in a microwave oven or toaster oven just long enough to soften the cheese and melt it slightly.

Makes 1 "A" (1 "B") satietizer serving.

SAVORY RICOTTA SNACKS

1 cup part-skim (low-fat) ricotta cheese
1 large egg
1 teaspoon finely chopped fresh parsley leaves
½ teaspoon dried instant minced onion
¼ teaspoon paprika
⅛ teaspoon dried oregano and/or dill leaves
12 whole wheat or plain melba toasts
2 tablespoons finely grated Parmesan cheese

In a medium-sized bowl, combine the ricotta, egg, parsley, instant onion, paprika, and herbs. Mix thoroughly. Refrigerate at
least 1 hour to let the flavors mingle. Spread one-fourth (one-
third) of the cheese mixture on 3 (4) melba toasts, then sprinkle
½ teaspoon of the grated cheese on each. Place under a preheated broiler for about 2 minutes or until topping is golden
and puffed. Serve immediately. 1 "A" serving = 3 snacks. (1
"B" serving = 4 snacks.)

Makes 4 "A" (3 "B") satietizer servings.

CHICKEN LIVERS WITH MUSHROOMS

1 tablespoon reduced-calorie margarine
1 medium-sized onion, thinly sliced
2 garlic cloves, minced
10 ounces [about ⅔ pound] chicken livers, rinsed and with all
    fat removed, cut into pieces
2 cups sliced fresh mushrooms
Salt and ground black pepper to taste

In a large skillet, melt the margarine over medium-high heat; then sauté the onion until very lightly browned. Add the garlic, liver pieces, and mushrooms and cook, stirring constantly, until the livers are barely pink inside. Season to taste.

Makes 4 "A" (3 "B") satietizer servings.

HERBED NEUFCHÂTEL CHEESE

6 ounces Neufchâtel cheese
¼ cup low-fat plain yogurt
2 tablespoons nonfat dry milk powder
1 tablespoon finely chopped chives or scallion greens
2 tablespoons finely chopped fresh parsley leaves
1 to 2 garlic cloves, finely minced
1 tablespoon finely minced shallots or onions (or scallion bottoms)
½ teaspoon each dried tarragon and basil leaves
¼ teaspoon dried dill or thyme leaves
Pinch of ground black pepper

TO SERVE:
Celery sticks, zucchini slices, cucumber slices, green pepper slices, and 2 to 3 plain crackers (per serving)

Beat the cheese with a wooden spoon (or an electric mixer or food processor) until soft; then beat in the yogurt and milk powder until very smooth. Add the remaining ingredients (quantities of the herbs and seasonings may be varied to taste), and mix thoroughly. Chill several hours to let the flavors mingle. The spread may be stored well wrapped in the refrigerator for up to a week. Serve with vegetables (as many as desired) and/or crackers.

Makes 4 "A" (3 "B") satietizer servings.

In-a-Minute Miniature Pizza

BASE:
½ *of a whole wheat or white English muffin or small loaf of pita (pocket) bread (A whole muffin or pita loaf should be split in half horizontally to make 2 circles; use 1 per serving.)*

CHEESE:
1 ounce (1¾ ounces) part-skim mozzarella cheese, grated
1 teaspoon (1½ teaspoons) grated Parmesan cheese

SAUCE:
2 tablespoons plain tomato sauce
¼ teaspoon dried oregano leaves
⅛ teaspoon dried basil leaves
Pinch of garlic powder OR ⅛ teaspoon finely chopped garlic

Toast the muffin or pita bread until lightly browned. Sprinkle the mozzarella cheese on top. Combine the sauce ingredients and drizzle over the mozzarella. Sprinkle the Parmesan on top. Heat in a toaster oven, conventional oven, or microwave oven until the cheese melts and is bubbly.

Makes 1 "A" (1 "B") satietizer serving.

The sauce ingredients may be multiplied for several servings and refrigerated up to 1 week in a covered container. For 1 [8-ounce] can tomato sauce, add 2 teaspoons oregano, 1 teaspoon basil, and ¼ teaspoon garlic powder. Use 2 tablespoons of sauce per serving.

MUSHROOM-WALNUT SPREAD

1 tablespoon reduced-calorie margarine
1 small onion, finely chopped
8 ounces fresh mushrooms, minced
⅛ teaspoon dried thyme leaves
Pinch of dried tarragon leaves
Pinch of ground sage
3 ounces [about ¾ cup] walnuts
1 hard-boiled large egg, shelled and coarsely chopped
2 tablespoons plain low-fat yogurt
Salt and ground black pepper to taste

> TO SERVE:
> *Celery sticks, zucchini slices, whole fresh mushrooms OR 1 rice*
>   *"cake" cracker (per serving)*

In a large skillet (preferably nonstick), melt the margarine over medium-high heat; then sauté the onion until tender. Add the mushrooms and herbs and continue sautéing until the mushrooms are tender. Cook until most (but not all) of the liquid has evaporated. Stir in the walnuts and egg and remove from the heat.

Stir in the yogurt. Purée the mixture in a food processor or food mill. Season to taste. Chill. The spread may be refrigerated up to 1 week. Adjust the seasonings, if necessary. Spread on raw vegetables (as many as desired) or a rice cake.

Makes 4 "A" (3 "B") satietizer servings.

Viennese Cheese Dumplings

1 *[12-ounce] container dry-curd cottage cheese*
1 *large egg yolk*
2½ *tablespoons dry Cream of Rice cereal or Cream of Wheat cereal*
1 *tablespoon sugar*
1 *teaspoon lemon juice*
¼ *cup fine crushed corn flake crumbs*

TO SERVE: (optional)
Unsweetened applesauce and ground cinnamon

If the cottage cheese contains large curds (or if smoother dumplings are desired), mash the cheese with a fork or put it through a sieve. Stir in the egg yolk, cereal, sugar, and lemon juice. Let the mixture stand for about 5 minutes.

Put the corn flake crumbs in a small bowl. Divide the cheese mixture into 12 equal portions. One at a time, spoon each portion into the crumbs, coat it, and form into a ball. (The crumbs should keep the cheese mixture from sticking to your hands.) Place the balls on a nonstick spray-coated baking sheet. Bake in a preheated 350°F oven for about 20 minutes or until quite firm. Serve the balls warm, at room temperature, or chilled. If desired, top each ball with 1 teaspoon applesauce and a pinch of cinnamon. 1 "A" serving = 3 balls. (1 "B" serving = 4 balls.)

Makes 4 "A" (3 "B") satietizer servings.

Spring Salad

½ cup (⅔ cup) 1% fat cottage cheese
2 tablespoons (3 tablespoons) commercial sour cream
1 to 2 scallions, including green tops, thinly sliced
1 small tomato, cored and diced
¼ cup diced cucumber
Salt and ground black pepper to taste

   TO SERVE:
Lettuce leaves (optional)

Combine salad ingredients and mix well. If desired, serve on a bed of lettuce.

Makes 1 "A" (1 "B") satietizer serving.

Instant Ricotta "Pudding"

⅓ cup (½ cup) part-skim low-fat ricotta cheese
2 tablespoons (3 tablespoons) low-fat plain yogurt
2 teaspoons (1 tablespoon) confectioner's sugar OR aspartame
   sweetener to taste
¼ teaspoon (generous ¼ teaspoon) vanilla extract
⅛ teaspoon (generous ⅛ teaspoon) orange extract (optional)
½ teaspoon grated orange rind (colored part only) (optional)

In a small bowl, combine all ingredients and mix until creamy. Serve immediately, or chill until serving time.

Makes 1 "A" (1 "B") satietizer serving.

Tuna in a Tomato "Flower"

1 *[6½-ounce] can water-packed tuna, drained and flaked*
2 *tablespoons reduced-calorie mayonnaise*
1 *stalk celery, finely chopped*
½ *teaspoon onion powder*
¼ *teaspoon dried dill weed*
4 *small (3 medium-sized) ripe, red tomatoes, cored*
2 *ounces grated cheese such as Swiss, mozzarella, muenster, or*
   colby

In a small bowl, combine the tuna, mayonnaise, celery, onion powder, and dill weed, and mix well. Use immediately or refrigerate, covered, for up to 4 days, and use as needed.

For each serving, cut 1 tomato into wedges from the top, leaving the wedges connected at the base of the tomato. Spread the wedges open like the petals of a flower and spoon one-fourth (one-third) of the tuna mixture into the center. Sprinkle ½ ounce (⅔ ounce) of the cheese on top. Heat in a microwave oven or under a heated broiler until the cheese melts.

Makes 4 "A" (3 "B") satietizer servings.

Peanut Butter Crackles

¼ *cup peanut butter*
2 *tablespoons packed brown sugar*
2 *tablespoons instant nonfat dry milk powder*
2 *tablespoons water*
⅛ *teaspoon ground cinnamon*
1 *cup ready-to-eat crispy rice cereal*

In a small saucepan, cook the peanut butter, sugar, milk powder, water, and cinnamon over medium-high heat. Stir constantly until the mixture is very hot and has thinned. Remove from the heat and stir in the cereal until completely mixed. Using about 1 tablespoon of the mixture for each, drop into 12 equal mounds on a plate. If desired, form into neat balls with your hands. Allow to set for about 10 minutes before serving. 1 "A" serving = 3 crackles (1 "B" serving = 4 crackles).

Makes 4 "A" (3 "B") satietizer servings.

WHOLE STUFFED ARTICHOKE

1 medium to large fresh artichoke
½ cup (⅔ cup) 1% fat cottage cheese
1½ tablespoons (2 tablespoons) reduced-calorie mayonnaise
2 tablespoons (3 tablespoons) chopped pimiento OR finely
*   chopped sweet red bell pepper*
½ to 1 teaspoon dried instant minced onion OR about 1 table-
*   spoon very finely chopped fresh onion*
½ teaspoon Worcestershire sauce
Pimiento strips for garnish (optional)

With a sharp knife, cut off the artichoke stem even with the base so the artichoke rests upright. Break off the row of small leaves around the base. Cut off about ¾ inch of the top of the leaf cone. Use kitchen shears or scissors to clip off the thorny tip of each leaf.

Put the artichoke in a small pot about half full of water. Cover the pot and bring to a boil over high heat. Reduce the heat and simmer the artichoke, covered, for 30 to 45 minutes or until it is very tender and a leaf pulls out easily. Drain the artichoke upside down and let it cool.

While the artichoke is cooking, prepare the stuffing. Combine the cottage cheese, mayonnaise, chopped pimiento (or red pepper), and onion. Add Worcestershire sauce and mix well. When the artichoke is ready, gently spread apart the center leaves and with a small spoon scrape out the tiny purple leaves and hairy choke. Fill the center of the artichoke with the cottage cheese mixture. If desired, garnish the top with strips of pimiento.

To eat the artichoke, pull off a leaf, dip it into the stuffing, and pull it through your teeth to scrape off the soft flesh inside. Continue with all the leaves until only the artichoke bottom remains. It is entirely edible.

Several artichokes may be cooked together ahead of time and then refrigerated until serving time. They are good chilled or at room temperature and may be stuffed a few hours before serving.

Makes 1 "A" (1 "B") satietizer serving.

RUMAKI

*6 whole chicken livers [about 1 ounce each], rinsed, each one
   separated into 2 lobes or sections*
12 canned water chestnuts, drained
6 slices bacon, cut in half crosswise
¼ cup soy sauce
Pinch of ground ginger

Fold a chicken liver piece around a water chestnut, wrap with a piece of bacon, and skewer on a round toothpick. Repeat to form 12 rumaki. Put the soy sauce and ginger in a bowl and add the rumaki. Turn to coat with the soy sauce mixture.

Let the rumaki marinate while the oven preheats to 425°F. Arrange them on a rack, set in a shallow pan, leaving room between them. Bake, turning them once, for about 10 minutes or until the bacon is crisp. Serve the rumaki warm or at room temperature. 1 "A" serving = 3 rumaki (1 "B" serving = 4 rumaki).

If preferred, the rumaki may be broiled about 6 inches from the heat source instead of baked.

Makes 4 "A" (3 "B") satietizer servings.

NUTTY POPCORN MIX

1½ cups popped popcorn prepared without oil (as in a hot air popper or microwave oven)
½ ounce—about 10 nuts (¾ ounce—about 15 nuts) shelled almonds, walnut halves, or peanuts
1 teaspoon finely grated Parmesan cheese
½ teaspoon garlic powder

Combine all ingredients and toss so the cheese and garlic powder are evenly distributed.

Makes 1 "A" (1 "B") satietizer serving.

SARDINE PUFF CANAPÉS

¼ cup reduced-calorie mayonnaise
3 tablespoons low-fat plain yogurt
1 [3¾-ounce] can sardines in tomato or mustard sauce, including sauce, mashed
1 large egg white
Pinch of cream of tartar
Finely chopped parsley leaves

   TO SERVE:
12 whole wheat melba toasts

In a medium-sized bowl, combine the mayonnaise and yogurt and mix well. Stir in the sardines until completely combined. In another bowl, beat the egg white with the cream of tartar until it forms stiff but not dry peaks. Fold the whites into the sardine mixture. For each serving, spread one-fourth (one-third) of the mixture on 3 (4) of the melba toasts. Sprinkle the tops lightly with parsley. Place under a preheated broiler for about 3 minutes or until lightly browned. Serve warm or at room temperature.

Makes 4 "A" (3 "B") satietizer servings.

Variation: For Sardine Dip, combine the mayonnaise, yogurt, and sardines as described above. Use the mixture as a dip for raw vegetables such as celery sticks, cucumber slices, raw mushrooms, or sliced green peppers.

Makes 4 "A" (3 "B") satietizer servings.

NACHOS WITH CHEESE

5 (7) small tortilla or nacho chips
¾ ounce (1 ounce) cheddar or longhorn cheese, cut into 5 (7) pieces
1 (1½) large black or green olive, cut into 5 (7) slices (optional)
5 (7) small pieces of hot (jalapeño) pepper or sweet green pepper (optional)

Top each chip with a 1 piece of cheese and, if desired, a slice of olive and piece of pepper. Heat the chips in a microwave oven or toaster oven or under the broiler just until the cheese is melted.

Makes 1 "A" (1 "B") satietizer serving.

Ricotta "Cheesecakes"

1⅓ cups part-skim (low-fat) ricotta cheese
1 large egg
2 large egg whites
2 tablespoons sugar
1 teaspoon vanilla extract
½ teaspoon lemon extract
4 medium-sized (3 large) fresh strawberries, sliced (optional)

Combine all the ingredients except the optional fruit in a food processor fitted with the steel blade or in a blender and process until smooth. Lightly coat 4 (3) ovenproof 6-ounce custard cups (or similar cups) with nonstick cooking spray and evenly divide the ricotta mixture among them. Set the cups in a larger pan and add boiling water to a depth of ½ inch. Bake the cheesecakes in a preheated 350°F oven for about 30 (35) minutes or until a small knife inserted in the center of one comes out almost clean. Remove the cups from the water and let the cheesecakes cool. Then cover and refrigerate them until cold and firm, at least 2 hours. (They may be refrigerated up to 4 days.) If desired, top each cheesecake with a sliced strawberry just before serving.

Makes 4 "A" (3 "B") satietizer servings.

SHERRIED CHICKEN LIVER PÂTÉ

1 tablespoon reduced-calorie margarine
1 medium-sized onion, finely chopped
1 garlic clove, minced
½ pound chicken livers, rinsed and all fat removed
1 cup sliced fresh mushrooms
¼ teaspoon salt (or to taste)
Pinch of ground black pepper (or to taste)
Pinch of ground thyme leaves
2 tablespoons dry sherry OR dry white wine
1 hard-boiled egg, coarsely chopped

TO SERVE:
Celery sticks and/or lettuce leaves (as desired)

In a large skillet, melt the margarine over medium-high heat; then sauté the onion until tender but not browned. Add the garlic, livers, mushrooms, salt, pepper, and thyme and continue cooking, stirring constantly, until the livers are cooked through. Add the sherry and hard-boiled egg and remove from the heat. Let the liver mixture cool slightly; then purée it with a food processor or food mill. Chill and adjust seasonings if necessary. Stuff in celery sticks or serve on a bed of lettuce.

Makes 4 "A" (3 "B") satietizer servings.

SALMON–CREAM CHEESE BALLS

1 [3-ounce] package cream cheese, softened
2 teaspoons dried instant minced onion OR 1 tablespoon very
*   finely chopped fresh onion*
2 teaspoons prepared white horseradish
1 teaspoon lemon juice
3½ ounces canned salmon [about ½ cup], drained
¼ cup finely chopped fresh parsley

   TO SERVE:
8 (9) whole wheat melba toasts

In a medium-sized bowl, combine thoroughly the cream cheese, onion, horseradish, and lemon juice. Stir in the salmon until evenly mixed. Chill the mixture until it can be handled; then with moistened hands, form it into 4 (3) equal-size balls. Roll the balls in the parsley to coat. Store in the refrigerator. Use 1 ball per serving and spread it on 2 (3) melba toasts per serving.

Makes 4 "A" (3 "B") satietizer servings.

15

Main Dishes—Meat

Swiss Steak Dinner with Vegetables

4 very lean cube steaks (1 pound total)
¾ cup beef bouillon made from a cube or powder
1 medium-sized onion, thinly sliced
½ to 1 teaspoon dried thyme leaves
⅛ teaspoon ground black pepper
1 teaspoon prepared mustard
½ cup plain tomato sauce
2 medium-sized carrots, cut into 2- by ½-inch sticks
2 stalks celery, cut into 2- by ½-inch sticks
1 cup sliced fresh mushrooms

TO SERVE:
4 ounces dry egg noodles, cooked

Coat a large skillet (preferably nonstick) with nonstick cooking spray, then preheat it over medium-high heat. Lightly brown the cube steaks on both sides and remove them to a platter. Drain

146

the skillet and wipe it out. Pour the bouillon into the skillet and bring it to a boil over medium-high heat. Add the onion and reduce the heat. Simmer, stirring occasionally, until the onion is limp. Stir in the thyme, pepper, mustard, and tomato sauce and heat to simmering. Add the cube steaks in one layer, turning them over once so the tops are coated with sauce. Scatter the carrots and celery around and over the meat. Cover the skillet tightly and simmer for 10 minutes. Add the mushrooms and baste the meat and vegetables with the sauce. Cook, covered, another 5 to 10 minutes or until the vegetables are tender but not mushy. Serve each cube steak topped with sauce and vegetables and accompanied with the hot, cooked noodles.

Makes 4 main-dish servings (1120); about 270 calories per serving (about 160 calories without noodles).

ORIENTAL BEEF AND BROCCOLI

SAUCE:
2 tablespoons soy sauce
2 tablespoons dry sherry
1 tablespoon water
1 garlic clove, minced
½ teaspoon honey
¼ teaspoon ground ginger

MEAT AND BROCCOLI:
1 pound very lean round steak, trimmed of all fat and slightly frozen for easier cutting
⅔ cup beef bouillon made from a cube or powder
1 medium-sized onion, thinly sliced
2½ cups fresh small broccoli florets and stem slices
2 scallions, including green tops, thinly sliced
1 tablespoon cornstarch
1 tablespoon cool water

TO SERVE:
2 cups hot cooked rice

In a medium-sized bowl, combine the sauce ingredients. Cut the steak across the grain into very thin (⅛- to ¼-inch-thick) slices about 2 inches long. Add the meat and toss to coat it. Set aside for 15 minutes, mixing occasionally.

In a very large, deep skillet or wok (preferably nonstick), bring the bouillon to a boil over medium-high heat. Add the onion, reduce the heat, and simmer, stirring often, until it is limp. Add the broccoli and scallions and cover the skillet. Steam for 5 minutes, or until the broccoli is crisp-tender. Using a slotted spoon, transfer the broccoli to a bowl. Add the meat and sauce to the juices in the skillet and cook over medium-high heat, stirring constantly, until the meat is just cooked through, about 3 minutes. In a small bowl, combine the cornstarch and water and add to the skillet. Cook, stirring, until the sauce thickens and boils. Return the broccoli to the skillet and cook, stirring until it is coated with sauce and heated through. Serve over the rice.

Makes 4 main-dish servings (1065); about 265 calories per serving (about 175 calories per serving without rice).

MARINATED FLANK STEAK WITH
VEGETABLE KEBABS

1 (1-pound) flank steak (or half of a 2-pound flank steak),
    trimmed of any surface fat
¼ cup soy sauce
¼ cup dry sherry
2 teaspoons vegetable oil
1 teaspoon sugar
2 garlic cloves, finely minced
½ teaspoon ground ginger
12 medium-sized fresh whole mushrooms
1 medium-sized zucchini, cut into 8 slices
8 frozen (dry pack) small white onions, thawed, OR 8 tiny
    white fresh onions, blanched and peeled
8 cherry tomatoes

Put the flank steak in a heavy, clear plastic storage bag. In a
small cup, combine the soy sauce, sherry, oil, sugar, garlic, and
ginger and mix thoroughly. Add to the bag and seal tightly with
a twist-tie, leaving a small air space. Rotate the bag to coat the
steak. (Alternatively, the steak may be marinated in a covered,
nonaluminum pan or dish.) Marinate the steak in the refrigerator for at least 1 hour or overnight, turning it occasionally.

Shortly before serving time, remove the steak from the refrigerator and let it come to room temperature. To assemble the
vegetable kebabs, using 4 skewers, slide a mushroom on the
skewer, then a slice of zucchini, then an onion (go across
the onion, rather than through the center), then a tomato. Repeat once and end with a third mushroom.

Drain the steak, reserving the marinade. Put the steak and
kebabs on a broiler rack set in a shallow pan and brush with
some of the reserved marinade. Broil about 5 inches below a
preheated broiler for 5 to 8 minutes on each side or until the
steak is cooked as desired (it is most tender and tasty when

served medium-rare; it can be tough when well done) and the vegetables are tender. Periodically brush the steak and vegetables with the marinade.

To serve, transfer the steak to a large cutting board or platter and cut it against the grain into very thin slices. Accompany each serving of steak with 1 vegetable kebab (vegetables may be removed from skewer, if desired). Heat any remaining marinade to boiling and offer with the steak and vegetables.

Makes 4 main-dish servings (1040); about 260 calories per serving.

GARDEN MINI MEAT LOAVES

1 pound extra-lean ground beef
¼ cup rolled oats
2 slices whole wheat bread, made into crumbs in a blender or food processor
1 (16-ounce) can tomatoes, drained
1 (10-ounce) package frozen chopped spinach, thawed and squeezed to remove all excess liquid
2 medium-sized carrots, grated or very finely chopped
1 large egg
1 tablespoon dried instant minced onion
1 teaspoon dried oregano leaves
½ teaspoon dried marjoram leaves
½ teaspoon salt
¼ teaspoon ground black pepper

In a medium-sized bowl, combine all ingredients and mix very well with your hands or a fork. Coat 12 standard-sized muffin cups with nonstick cooking spray, then pack the meat mixture evenly into each cup, heaping it slightly if necessary. Place the muffin cups on a baking sheet to catch drippings. Bake in a preheated 350°F oven for 40 to 45 minutes or until the meat loaves are browned on top and cooked through. Remove immediately to a serving dish.

Makes 6 main-dish servings (1325); about 220 calories per serving.

CHILI CON CARNE

The calories for the ground beef are lower than in some recipes because the fat released during cooking is drained off.

¾ pound extra-lean ground beef
1 medium-sized onion, finely chopped
2 garlic cloves, minced
2 medium-sized carrots, grated
3 stalks celery, finely chopped
1 (16-ounce) can tomatoes, finely chopped, including juice
1 (8-ounce) can plain tomato sauce
1 (15- to 16-ounce) can dark kidney beans, drained
1 tablespoon plain or red wine vinegar
1 to 2 tablespoons chili powder (or to taste)

In a large, deep skillet (preferably nonstick), brown the ground beef over medium-high heat, breaking it with a fork. As it browns, add the onion and garlic. When the meat has browned and the onion is tender, spoon off and discard the fat. Add the remaining ingredients, and mix thoroughly. Cover loosely, reduce the heat, and simmer, stirring occasionally, for 30 to 40 minutes or until the sauce has thickened and the flavors have mingled. If the sauce is still too thin, remove the cover and boil it down for a few minutes, stirring often.

Makes 4 main-dish servings (1090); about 270 calories per serving.

SWEET-AND-SOUR GROUND BEEF AND CABBAGE

Here's a quick and easy variation on Eastern European stuffed cabbage.

The calories for the ground beef are lower than in some recipes because the fat released during cooking is drained off.

1 pound extra-lean ground beef
1 medium-sized onion, finely chopped
2 garlic cloves, minced
1 (15- to 16-ounce) can plain tomato sauce
¼ cup unsweetened applesauce
¼ cup water
3 tablespoons apple cider vinegar
1 tablespoon dark brown sugar
⅛ teaspoon dried thyme leaves
Pinch of ground black pepper
4½ cups (about 1 pound) shredded green (white) cabbage

In a large, deep skillet (preferably nonstick), brown the ground beef over medium-high heat, breaking it with a fork. As it browns, add the onion and garlic. When the meat has browned and the onion is tender, spoon off and discard the fat. Add the tomato sauce, applesauce, water, vinegar, brown sugar, thyme, and pepper. Bring the mixture to a boil, stirring constantly. Stir in the cabbage. Reduce the heat and simmer, covered, stirring occasionally, for 20 to 25 minutes or until the cabbage is very tender. If the sauce is too thin, boil it down for a few minutes, stirring constantly.

Makes 4 main-dish servings (980);
about 245 calories per serving.

CURRIED BEEF, CHICK-PEAS, AND CAULIFLOWER

The calories for the ground beef are lower than in some recipes because the fat released during cooking is drained off.

½ pound extra-lean ground beef
1 small onion, finely chopped
1 (16-ounce) can tomatoes, including juice, finely chopped
1 (15- to 16-ounce) can chick-peas, drained
3 cups small fresh cauliflower florets
1 teaspoon curry powder (or to taste)
1 bay leaf, crumbled
⅛ teaspoon ground black pepper

TO SERVE:
2 cups hot cooked rice

In a large, deep skillet (preferably nonstick), brown the ground
beef over medium-high heat, breaking it with a fork. As it
browns, add the onion. When the meat has browned and the
onion is tender, spoon off and discard the fat. Add the tomatoes
and their juice, chick-peas, cauliflower, curry powder, bay leaf,
and pepper. Reduce the heat, cover the skillet, and simmer, stirring occasionally, for about 20 minutes or until the cauliflower
is almost tender. Remove the cover and continue simmering,
stirring frequently, for 5 to 10 minutes longer or until the sauce
is the desired thickness. Serve over the rice.

Makes 4 main-dish servings (1245);
about 310 calories per serving (about 220 calories per serving
without rice).

BEEF AND VEGETABLE SKILLET

The calories for the ground beef are lower than in some recipes because the fat released during cooking is drained off.

¾ pound extra-lean ground beef
1 cup beef bouillon made from cubes or powder
1 medium-sized onion, finely chopped
3 stalks celery, thinly sliced
1 (16-ounce) can tomatoes, including juice, coarsely chopped
1 cup frozen loose-pack corn kernels
2 medium-sized green peppers, thinly sliced
1 teaspoon chili powder
1 cup dry instant precooked rice

In a large, deep skillet (preferably nonstick), brown the ground beef over medium-high heat, breaking it with a fork. When the meat has browned, spoon off and discard the fat. Add the bouillon and bring it to a boil. Stir in the onion and celery, reduce the heat, and simmer, stirring often, until the vegetables are just tender. Stir in the tomatoes and their juice, corn kernels, green peppers, and chili powder. Bring to a simmer, stirring, and cook for 2 to 3 minutes or until the corn and pepper are just tender. Stir in the rice, cover tightly, and remove from the heat. Let stand 5 minutes; then fluff with a fork.

Makes 4 main-dish servings (1150); about 285 calories per serving.

16

Main Dishes—Poultry

CHICKEN IN ORANGE SAUCE

4 chicken breast halves or 8 small drumsticks (about 2 pounds),
*   skin and fat removed*
⅔ cup orange juice
½ teaspoon grated orange peel (colored part only)
1 chicken bouillon cube or envelope of powder
Pinch of ground black pepper
Pinch of ground ginger
1 tablespoon cornstarch
1 tablespoon water
2 scallions, including green tops, thinly sliced on the diagonal
1 medium-sized navel orange, peeled and sectioned

Coat a large skillet with nonstick cooking spray and preheat it over medium-high heat. Lightly brown the chicken pieces on both sides. In a small cup, combine the orange juice, peel,

155

bouillon cube or powder, pepper, and ginger. Pour over the chicken. Arrange the chicken flesh side down in the juice. Bring the juice to a boil, reduce the heat, cover the skillet, and gently simmer for about 45 minutes or until the chicken is tender. If breasts are used, slide them around occasionally to make sure they don't stick. If drumsticks are used, turn them occasionally. Using tongs or a slotted spoon, transfer the chicken pieces to a serving platter.

In a small cup, combine the cornstarch and water and add to the juices in the skillet, along with the scallions. Cook, stirring constantly, until the sauce thickens and just comes to a boil. Stir in the orange sections. Spoon the sauce over the chicken pieces.

Makes 4 main-dish servings (685); about 170 calories per serving.

BROILED HERBED CHICKEN BREASTS

*4 medium-sized chicken breast halves (about 2 pounds), skin removed**
1 tablespoon vegetable oil
2 tablespoons red wine vinegar
¼ teaspoon dried rosemary leaves, crushed
¼ teaspoon dried thyme leaves
¼ teaspoon dried tarragon leaves
Pinch of paprika
Pinch of black pepper

Coat a broiler pan or baking pan with nonstick cooking spray. Arrange the chicken pieces in the pan with the bone side up. Broil about 6 inches from the heat source for about 20 minutes. Meanwhile, combine the remaining ingredients in a small bowl and mix well. Turn the pieces over and brush them with about half the herb mixture. Continue broiling (brushing once with the remaining herb mixture) for 10 to 15 minutes or until the chicken juices run clear when pricked with a fork.

* (Note: If desired, 8 chicken drumsticks may be substituted for the breasts. Brush them on all sides with the herb mixture and turn them several times during the broiling period. Broil for a total of about 20 to 25 minutes or until done. 2 drumsticks = 1 serving.)

Makes 4 main-dish servings (625); about 155 calories per serving.

OVEN-BARBECUED CHICKEN

BARBECUE SAUCE:
1 (8-ounce) can plain tomato sauce
⅓ cup apple cider vinegar
1 tablespoon Worcestershire sauce
1 tablespoon reduced-calorie margarine
2 tablespoons packed dark brown sugar
1 tablespoon dried instant minced onion
2 garlic cloves, finely minced
½ teaspoon powdered mustard
½ teaspoon salt
¼ teaspoon hot red pepper sauce
1 bay leaf

CHICKEN:
1½ pounds chicken breasts and/or drumsticks, skin and fat removed

Combine the sauce ingredients in a small saucepan and bring to a boil over medium-high heat. Reduce the heat and simmer, stirring occasionally, for 15 minutes. Discard the bay leaf. Cool the sauce and store it in the refrigerator until needed. (It may be refrigerated up to 4 days or frozen for longer storage.)

Line a 9- by 13-inch (or similar) baking dish with aluminum foil or coat it with nonstick cooking spray. Pour about half of the prepared barbecue sauce in the bottom of the pan. Arrange the chicken pieces in the sauce, then pour the remaining sauce on top. Bake, covered, in a preheated 350°F oven for 30 minutes. Then remove the cover, and bake about 30 minutes longer, basting often, until the chicken is tender and the sauce has thickened and coated the pieces. If the sauce seems to be drying out too much, add a few tablespoons of water.

Makes 6 main-dish servings (1010); about 170 calories per serving.

CHICKEN CACCIATORE

6 chicken breast halves, skinned and boned (about 1½ pounds)
¼ cup dry white wine
1 medium-sized onion, thinly sliced
2 medium-sized green peppers, thinly sliced
2 cups sliced fresh mushrooms
2 garlic cloves, minced
1 (16-ounce) can tomatoes, including juice, coarsely chopped
1 teaspoon dried oregano leaves
1 teaspoon dried basil leaves
¼ teaspoon dried rosemary leaves, crushed
⅛ teaspoon ground black pepper
½ cup canned tomato paste
6 ounces dry spaghetti, cooked

Coat a large, deep skillet with nonstick cooking spray and preheat it over medium-high heat. Lightly brown the chicken breasts on both sides. Add the wine and cook for 2 minutes. With tongs or slotted spoon, remove the chicken breasts to a platter.

Add the onion to the skillet, reduce the heat, and simmer until it is limp. Add the green peppers, mushrooms, garlic, tomatoes and their juice, herbs, and black pepper. Bring the mixture to a simmer, stirring occasionally. Return the chicken breasts to the skillet, burying them in the sauce. Cover and simmer until the chicken is cooked through and tender, about 25 minutes.

Remove the chicken pieces to a platter. Stir the tomato paste into the juices in the skillet. Bring the sauce to a simmer, stirring. Return the chicken to the skillet and baste it with the sauce. Serve over cooked spaghetti.

Any leftover chicken in sauce can be refrigerated or frozen and reheated; spaghetti, however, should be freshly cooked as needed.

Makes 6 main-dish servings (1765); about 295 calories per serving (about 190 calories per serving without spaghetti).

CHINESE-STYLE CHICKEN AND VEGETABLES

¾ cup chicken bouillon made from a cube or powder
2 teaspoons soy sauce
1 medium-sized onion, thinly sliced
2 stalks celery, thinly sliced on the diagonal
1 pound skinned and boned raw chicken breast, trimmed of fat
  and cut into 1-inch pieces
2 cups thinly sliced fresh mushrooms
1 medium-sized green pepper, cut into 1-inch squares
2 cups fresh snow peas, trimmed and strings removed, OR
  2 cups small broccoli florets and stem slices
⅛ teaspoon ground ginger (or to taste)
1 cup fresh mung bean sprouts
1 tablespoon cornstarch
2 tablespoons cool water

TO SERVE:
2 cups hot cooked rice

In a large skillet or wok (preferably nonstick), bring the broth and soy sauce to a simmer over medium-high heat, add the onion and celery, and cook, stirring frequently, for about 3 minutes. Add the chicken and cook, stirring frequently, until the pieces are opaque and cooked through. Add the mushrooms, pepper, snow peas or broccoli, and ginger. Cover the skillet and steam for about 3 minutes or until the green vegetables are crisp-tender. Add the bean sprouts and cook, stirring, for 1 to 2 minutes longer. (For best taste, do not overcook!) In a small cup, thoroughly mix the cornstarch and water. Add to the skillet and stir constantly until sauce thickens and becomes translucent. Serve immediately over the rice.

Makes 4 main-dish servings (1130); about 280 calories per serving (about 190 calories per serving without rice).

QUICK PROVINCIAL CHICKEN SKILLET

1 *pound skinned and boned raw chicken breast meat, trimmed of fat and cut into 2-inch by ½-inch strips*
2 *tablespoons reduced-calorie margarine*
1 *medium-sized onion, thinly sliced*
2 *garlic cloves, minced*
2 *medium-sized zucchini (about 1 pound), stem ends trimmed and thinly sliced*
1 *medium-sized yellow squash (about 8 ounces), stem end trimmed and thinly sliced*
1 *cup sliced fresh mushrooms*
1 *(16-ounce) can tomatoes, drained and coarsely chopped*
½ *teaspoon dried basil leaves*
½ *teaspoon dried thyme leaves*
¼ *teaspoon dried oregano leaves*
⅛ *teaspoon ground black pepper*
5 *large black olives, pitted*
1 *tablespoon lemon juice*

Coat a large skillet (preferably nonstick) with nonstick cooking spray and preheat it over medium-high heat. Add the chicken and cook, stirring constantly, for about 3 minutes or until just cooked through. Transfer to a serving dish.

In the same skillet, melt the margarine, add the onion and garlic, and sauté about 1 minute or until limp. Add the zucchini, yellow squash, and mushrooms and continue sautéing for 3 to 5 minutes or until the squash is crisp-tender. Return the chicken to the skillet along with the tomatoes, herbs, pepper, olives and lemon juice. Cook, stirring constantly, until the mixture is completely heated through.

Makes 4 main-dish servings (970); about 240 calories per serving.

GINGERED CHICKEN SALAD (IN PITA)

⅓ cup low-fat plain yogurt
2½ tablespoons reduced-calorie mayonnaise
1 medium-sized carrot, grated
2 teaspoons honey
2 teaspoons apple cider vinegar
⅛ teaspoon ground ginger
1⅔ cups diced, cooked chicken breast meat
1 medium-sized ripe pear, cored and diced
½ cup halved seedless grapes
2 stalks celery, diced
1 tablespoon hulled sunflower seeds

TO SERVE (optional):
*4 small whole wheat loaves of pita (pocket) bread OR 4 large
lettuce leaves*

In a medium-sized bowl, combine the yogurt, mayonnaise, carrot, honey, vinegar, and ginger and mix well to make a dressing. Add the remaining salad ingredients and toss gently until completely coated. Chill at least 1 hour to let flavors mingle. To serve, cut open the top of each pita and fill with one-fourth of the chicken salad. Or, if desired, mound each serving on a lettuce leaf.

Makes 4 main-dish servings (1130); about 280 calories per serving with pita bread (about 200 calories per serving without pita).

Turkey Normandy

1 pound thinly sliced raw turkey breast cutlets (6 to 8 cutlets)
Ground black pepper
⅔ cup apple juice or cider
1 teaspoon butter-flavored granules
1 small onion, finely chopped
2 stalks celery, thinly sliced
1 large, firm apple (such as a Granny Smith or Winesap), un-
*   peeled, cored and thinly sliced*
1 tablespoon raisins
1 tablespoon cornstarch
½ cup low-fat plain yogurt

Sprinkle the turkey breast cutlets lightly with black pepper. Coat a large nonstick skillet with nonstick cooking spray and preheat it over medium-high heat. Cook the cutlets about 3 minutes on each side or until they are just cooked through. To keep the cutlets tender, be sure not to overcook them. Transfer the turkey to a platter.

In the same skillet, bring the apple juice to a boil. Scrape up and stir in any brown bits from the bottom of the skillet. Add the butter-flavored granules and stir until they are dissolved. Stir in the onion, celery, apple, and raisins and simmer until all are tender, about 5 minutes. Stir the cornstarch into the yogurt and add to the skillet. Cook, stirring constantly, until the sauce thickens and just comes to a boil. Remove from the heat. Return the cutlets to the skillet and push them under the sauce. Serve with sauce on top.

Makes 4 main-dish servings (875); about 220 calories per serving.

Turkey with Wine and Mushrooms

1 pound thinly sliced raw turkey breast cutlets (6 to 8 cutlets)
Ground black pepper
½ cup chicken bouillon made from a cube or powder
1 medium-sized onion, very thinly sliced
2 cups thinly sliced fresh mushrooms
1 medium-sized green pepper, thinly sliced
2 stalks celery, thinly sliced
¼ cup dry white wine
½ teaspoon dried thyme leaves
¼ teaspoon dried basil leaves
1 tablespoon cornstarch
1 tablespoon cool water
1 tablespoon finely chopped fresh parsley

Sprinkle the turkey breast cutlets lightly with black pepper. Coat a large nonstick skillet with nonstick cooking spray and preheat it over medium-high heat. Cook the cutlets about 3 minutes on each side or until they are just cooked through. To keep the cutlets tender, be sure not to overcook them. Transfer the turkey to a platter.

In the same skillet, bring the bouillon to a boil. Scrape up and stir in any brown bits from the bottom of the skillet. Add the onion, reduce the heat, and simmer a few minutes, stirring occasionally, until it is limp. Add the mushrooms, green pepper, celery, wine, thyme, and basil. Simmer, stirring, until the vegetables are just tender. Dissolve the cornstarch in the water and add to the skillet. Cook, stirring, until the sauce thickens and just comes to a boil. Return the cutlets to the skillet and push them under the sauce. Serve with some of the sauce. Sprinkle the parsley on top.

Makes 4 main-dish servings (725); about 180 calories per serving.

TURKEY-SPROUT WALDORF SALAD

¼ cup low-fat plain yogurt
2 tablespoons reduced-calorie mayonnaise
2 tablespoons orange or apple juice
1½ cups diced cooked turkey breast meat
1½ cups fresh mung bean sprouts
1 medium-sized unpeeled apple, cored and diced
2 stalks celery, diced
2 tablespoons raisins
2 tablespoons walnut pieces

   TO SERVE:
8 ounces very fresh raw spinach, well rinsed, drained, and stems
   trimmed

In a medium-sized bowl, combine the yogurt, mayonnaise, and orange or apple juice. Stir in the remaining salad ingredients and toss gently until completely coated. Chill at least 1 hour to let flavors mingle. To serve, mound on a bed of raw spinach.

                    Makes 4 main-dish servings (865);
about 215 calories per serving.

17

Main Dishes—
Fish and Shellfish

CREOLE-STYLE FISH DINNER

1 tablespoon reduced-calorie margarine
1 medium-sized onion, thinly sliced
1 large green pepper, thinly sliced
2 stalks celery, thinly sliced
1 (16-ounce) can tomatoes, including juice, coarsely chopped
½ teaspoon dried thyme leaves
½ teaspoon dried basil leaves
⅛ teaspoon hot red pepper sauce (or to taste)
1 pound skinless fish fillets, such as flounder, sole, cod, or had-
  dock
1 (8-ounce) can plain tomato sauce

TO SERVE:
2 cups hot cooked rice

In a large, deep skillet (preferably nonstick), melt the margarine over medium-high heat. Add the onion and sauté until tender. And the green pepper and celery and sauté 1 to 2 minutes longer. Stir in the tomatoes and their juice, thyme, basil, and pepper sauce. Heat to simmering, stirring. Lay the fish fillets on top of the sauce. Cover the skillet and steam the fish for about 5 to 10 minutes (depending on the thickness of the fillets), or just until the fish becomes opaque. With a slotted spoon, remove the fish and vegetables to a serving plate. Add the tomato sauce to the skillet, raise the heat, and quickly boil down the sauce to the desired thickness. Spoon the sauce over the fish and serve over the rice.

Makes 4 main-dish servings (1000); about 250 calories per serving (about 160 calories per serving without rice).

LAYERED SOLE CASSEROLE

1 (10-ounce) package frozen chopped spinach, thawed and squeezed to remove excess liquid
2 tablespoons reduced-calorie margarine
1 pound skinless sole or flounder fillets
1 (16-ounce can) tomatoes, drained and chopped
1 teaspoon dried basil leaves
½ teaspoon dried thyme leaves
Pinch of ground black pepper
1 small red onion, very thinly sliced into rings
1 medium-sized green pepper, thinly sliced into rings

Spread the spinach in an even layer in the bottom of a 7- by 11-inch (or similar) baking dish. Dab with 1 tablespoon of the margarine. Arrange the fish in a single layer over the spinach. Cover the fish with the tomatoes, then sprinkle with the herbs and black pepper. Arrange the onion and pepper rings attractively on top. Dab the remaining 1 tablespoon margarine over all. Cover the casserole and bake it in a 400°F oven for 20 to 25 minutes or until the fish is cooked through.

Makes 4 main-dish servings (555); about 140 calories per serving.

POACHED TURBOT WITH MIREPOIX SAUCE

Mirepoix is the French word for an aromatic and colorful mixture of diced onion, carrots, and celery sautéed together. In this recipe, the mirepoix enhances both the flavor and appearance of a rich-tasting sauce.

If desired, the fish may be topped with a simple mirepoix that is not made into a sauce (that is, does not have the flour, milk powder, and hot water added to it). This fish dinner would then have a mere 130 calories per serving.

FOR THE SAUCE:
2 tablespoons reduced-calorie margarine
1 cup finely diced carrot
¾ cup finely diced celery
½ cup finely diced onion
¼ teaspoon dried basil leaves
¼ teaspoon dried marjoram leaves
2 tablespoons all-purpose flour
⅓ cup instant nonfat dry milk powder
1 cup hot water
Salt and ground black pepper to taste

FOR THE FISH:

1½ cups water
¼ cup white wine vinegar
⅛ teaspoon ground black pepper
1 bay leaf
1 pound skinless turbot or flounder fillets (or similar fish)

For the sauce, melt the margarine in a medium-sized saucepan over medium-high heat. Add the carrot, celery, onion, basil, and marjoram and cook, stirring constantly, for about 5 minutes or until the carrot is crisp-tender. Stir in the flour, then the milk powder. Slowly pour in the hot water, stirring constantly to avoid lumps. As soon as the sauce thickens and comes to a boil, reduce the heat and simmer for 2 minutes, stirring frequently. Adjust the seasonings to taste. Cover the sauce and leave it over very low heat while you poach the fish. Stir occasionally so a "skin" does not form on top.

To poach the fish, combine the water, vinegar, pepper, and bay leaf in a large, deep skillet. Bring to a boil over medium-high heat, then reduce to a simmer. Add the fish fillets in one layer or slightly overlapping and bring back to a simmer. Simmer very gently for 3 to 5 minutes or until the fish becomes opaque. (Do not overcoook or the fillets may fall apart.) Carefully remove the fillets with a slotted, flat pancake turner, draining them very well, and put them on a serving platter. Spoon the warm sauce over the fillets and serve immediately.

Makes 4 main-dish servings (650); about 160 calories per serving.

SOLE AND ASPARAGUS BUNDLES

¾ pound fresh asparagus OR 1 (8-ounce) package frozen aspar-
    agus spears
1 pound small skinless sole or flounder fillets
⅓ cup Italian-style dry bread crumbs
3 tablespoons reduced-calorie margarine

If using fresh asparagus, trim the ends and cut into 6-inch pieces. Cook in a small amount of boiling water for about 5 minutes or until crisp-tender. If using frozen asparagus, thaw it completely. In a pinch, drained canned asparagus may be substituted, but it does not have the same taste or texture as fresh or frozen asparagus.

Lay out the fish fillets with the skinned side facing up. Lay the asparagus spears across the center of each fillet so the ends stick over the sides. Sprinkle the asparagus with 2 tablespoons of the bread crumbs and dot with 1 tablespoon of the margarine. Roll up each fillet around the asparagus and arrange in a nonstick spray-coated baking dish so they will not unroll. Sprinkle with the remaining bread crumbs and dot with the remaining margarine.

Cover the dish tightly with aluminum foil and bake in a preheated 400°F oven for 15 to 20 minutes or until the fish just flakes when touched with a fork. Or, if desired, cover the dish with heavy-duty plastic wrap and bake in a microwave oven on high power, rotating the dish occasionally, for about 6 minutes or until done as indicated above.

Makes 4 main-dish servings (650); about 160 calories per serving.

HEARTY NEW ENGLAND–STYLE FISH CHOWDER

3 cups potatoes peeled and diced in ½-inch cubes
2 stalks celery, diced
1 medium-sized onion, finely chopped
2⅔ cups water
2 vegetable or chicken bouillon cubes or envelopes of powder
2 teaspoons butter-flavored granules
1½ pounds skinless cod or haddock fillets, cut into 1-inch
  pieces OR whole bay or sea scallops
⅓ cup instant nonfat dry milk powder
¼ cup instant mashed potato flakes
⅛ to ¼ teaspoon ground black pepper

In a 3-quart or similar saucepan, combine the potatoes, celery, onion, 2 cups of the water, and bouillon cubes or powder. Bring to a boil, covered over high heat, reduce the heat and simmer for 15 minutes. Stir in the butter-flavored granules until dissolved. Add the fish (or scallops) and bring back to a simmer. Cook for 5 to 8 minutes longer, or until the fish pieces (or scallops) are opaque and the potatoes are just tender. Dissolve the milk powder in the remaining ⅔ cup water and stir into the chowder. Bring back to a simmer and stir in the potato flakes to thicken the broth. Season to taste with the pepper.

Makes 6 main-dish servings (1080); 180 calories per serving.

VARIATION: Use only 1 pound fish or scallops.

Makes 4 generous servings (900); 225 calories per serving.

Zucchini Halves Stuffed with Tuna

2 medium-sized zucchini (about 8 ounces each)
½ cup chicken bouillon made from a cube or powder
1 small onion, finely chopped
1 stalk celery, finely chopped
½ teaspoon dried thyme leaves
⅛ teaspoon black pepper
1 (6½-ounce) can water-packed tuna, drained and flaked
¼ cup Italian-style dry bread crumbs
2 tablespoons finely grated Parmesan cheese

Trim the stem end from each zucchini and cut in half lengthwise. Use a melon baller or small knife to scoop the flesh from the inside of each half, leaving a ¼-inch-thick shell. Chop the flesh and set it aside with the shells.

In a large skillet, bring the bouillon to a boil over medium-high heat; add the onion and celery. Reduce the heat and simmer, stirring frequently, until the onion is translucent and tender. Add the chopped zucchini, thyme, and pepper and cook, stirring constantly, for about 2 minutes or until most, but not all, of the liquid has evaporated. Remove from the heat and stir in the tuna and bread crumbs. If the mixture is very dry, add a bit of bouillon or water. Stuff the zucchini with the mixture, heaping it in the center. Sprinkle the cheese on top.

Wash the skillet; then return it to the heat. Add water to a depth of about ¼ inch. Place the stuffed zucchini in the skillet, being sure that the water level is not higher than the sides of the shells. Bring the water to a simmer, cover the skillet, and steam the stuffed zucchini for about 10 minutes or until the shells are tender when pierced with the tip of a knife.

Makes 2 main-dish servings (465);
about 230 calories per serving.

BAKED POTATOES WITH TUNA FLORENTINE TOPPING

*4 medium-sized (about 6 ounces each) baking potatoes, such as
    Idaho or russet*
1 tablespoon reduced-calorie margarine
1 medium-sized onion, finely chopped
1 garlic clove, minced
1 (16-ounce) can tomatoes, including juice, coarsely chopped
*1 (10-ounce) package frozen chopped spinach, thawed and
    drained*
1 teaspoon dried basil leaves
½ teaspoon dried marjoram leaves
⅛ teaspoon ground black pepper
*2 (6½-ounce) cans water-packed tuna, drained and broken into
    large flakes*
4 teaspoons grated Parmesan cheese

Scrub the potatoes well and pierce them with a fork; then bake
them in a conventional or microwave oven until tender.

Meanwhile, melt the margarine in a large skillet (preferably
nonstick) over medium-high heat. Add the onion and garlic and
sauté until tender. Stir in the tomatoes and their juice, spinach,
basil, marjoram, and black pepper. Cook, stirring often, for
about 15 minutes or until most, but not all, of the liquid has
evaporated. Gently stir in the tuna and cook until it is just
heated through.

To serve, cut each hot baked potato in half and fluff the flesh
with a fork. Top with one-fourth of the tuna-spinach mixture.
Sprinkle 1 teaspoon cheese over each serving.

Makes 4 servings (1145);
about 285 calories per serving (about 175 calories per serving
without baked potatoes).

MOLDED SALMON-CUCUMBER SALAD

This light and delicate salad makes a very nice luncheon dish. If molded into an attractive shape and served in smaller portions, it could also be an elegant first course for a company dinner.

2 tablespoons lemon juice
1 envelope unflavored gelatin
½ cup boiling water
1 chicken or vegetable bouillon cube, crumbled, OR 1 envelope
    of powder
1 (7¾-ounce or similar) can pink salmon, drained
1 cup peeled and coarsely chopped cucumber
2 scallions, including green tops, finely chopped
½ cup low-fat plain yogurt
¼ cup reduced-calorie mayonnaise
2 tablespoons chopped fresh parsley leaves
1 teaspoon dried dill weed
¼ teaspoon powdered mustard

    TO SERVE:
Large lettuce leaves for platter
1 large cucumber, peeled in strips and sliced

Put the lemon juice in a small bowl and sprinkle the gelatin on top to soften it. Add the boiling water and bouillon cube or powder and stir until the gelatin and bouillon are dissolved. Put the remaining ingredients in a food processor fitted with the steel blade or in a blender and add the gelatin mixture. Process until almost puréed. Pour into a 3½- to 4-cup mold that has been lightly coated with nonstick cooking spray. Chill several hours or until the salad is completely set. (It may be made up to 2 days ahead.) Run a knife around the edge of the salad and unmold it onto a bed of lettuce. Surround it with the cucumber slices. To eat, spread some of the salad on cucumber slices (or on crackers—add the calories for the crackers).

Makes 3 main-dish servings (675); about 225 calories per serving. (Makes 8 hors d'oeuvre servings; about 85 calories each.)

SEAFOOD EGG FOU YONG

3 large eggs
2 large egg whites
1 cup (canned or fresh) cooked tiny shrimp OR pieces of crab-meat
1 cup fresh mung bean sprouts
1 stalk celery, diced
¼ cup thinly sliced scallions, including green tops, OR diced yellow onion
¼ cup thinly sliced fresh or drained canned mushrooms
¼ teaspoon salt
Pinch of ground black pepper

SAUCE: (optional)
2 teaspoons cornstarch
⅔ cup cool water
1 teaspoon soy sauce
½ of a chicken or vegetable bouillon cube or envelope of powder

TO SERVE: (optional)
1½ cups hot cooked rice

Put the eggs and egg whites in a medium-sized bowl and beat with a fork until well mixed. Stir in the shrimp, bean sprouts, celery, scallions or onion, mushrooms, salt, and pepper. Preheat a 10-inch nonstick skillet over medium-high heat and coat it with nonstick cooking spray. Add the egg mixture and spread it evenly in the skillet. Cook over medium to medium-high heat until the bottom of the egg fou yong is firm; then divide it into three even pieces with a pancake turner. Turn over each piece and cook on the second side for a few minutes until done.

While the egg fou yong is cooking, make the sauce if desired. Put the cornstarch in a small saucepan; slowly add the water while stirring. Add the remaining ingredients and put the saucepan over medium-high heat. Cook, stirring constantly, until the mixture thickens slightly and comes to a boil. Just before serving, spoon some of the warm sauce over the egg fou yong. If desired, accompany with ½ cup rice per serving.

Makes 3 main-dish servings (775); about 260 calories per serving with sauce and rice (about 170 calories per serving without rice).

Linguine with White Scallop Sauce

¼ cup water
¼ cup finely chopped onion
1 garlic clove, finely minced
2 teaspoons butter-flavored granules
2 tablespoons finely chopped fresh parsley leaves
1 teaspoon dried tarragon leaves
1 teaspoon dried chives OR 2 teaspoons chopped fresh chives
¼ cup dry white wine
2 cups sliced fresh mushrooms
Pinch each of salt and ground black pepper
1 pound small bay scallops OR large bay scallops, cut into
*   fourths*
1½ tablespoons cornstarch
1 tablespoon grated Parmesan cheese
¾ cup low-fat plain yogurt
4 ounces dry spinach linguine or regular linguine, cooked according to the package directions

In a medium-sized saucepan, bring the water to a boil over medium-high heat; add the onion, garlic, and butter-flavored granules. Reduce the heat and simmer, stirring frequently, until the onion is tender and most of the water has evaporated. If the water evaporates too soon, add a few tablespoons more. Stir in the parsley, tarragon, chives, wine, mushrooms, salt, and pepper. Simmer for 1 minute; then add the scallops. Cook, stirring frequently, for about 3 minutes or until the scallops become opaque. (Do not overcook the scallops or they may become tough.) Stir the cornstarch and Parmesan cheese into the yogurt and add to the saucepan while stirring. Cook, stirring, just until the sauce comes to a boil. Toss the scallop sauce with the warm linguine.

Makes 4 main-dish servings (1105); about 275 calories per serving (about 170 calories per serving without linguine).

Pasta with Sherried Shrimp

¼ cup dry sherry
½ cup chicken bouillon made from a cube or powder
1 tablespoon lemon juice
2 teaspoons butter-flavored granules
2 tablespoons chopped scallions, including green tops
1 pound fresh or frozen small shrimp, shelled and deveined
1 tablespoon cornstarch
1 tablespoon cool water
¼ cup chopped fresh parsley leaves
4 ounces dry fettuccine or spaghetti, cooked

In a large skillet, combine the sherry, bouillon, and lemon juice. Bring to a boil over medium-high heat. Add the butter-flavored granules, reduce the heat, and simmer, stirring, until they are dissolved. Add the scallions and shrimp and simmer about 3 to 5 minutes longer or until the shrimp are opaque. Stir together the cornstarch and water and add to the skillet. Cook, stirring constantly, until the sauce thickens and comes to a boil. Remove from the heat and stir in the parsley. Toss the sauce with the hot cooked pasta.

Makes 4 main-dish servings (930); about 230 calories per serving (about 125 calories per serving without pasta).

CRAB AND RICE SALAD

SALAD:
12 ounces fresh cooked crabmeat, picked over, OR 2 (6-ounce packages) frozen crabmeat, thawed, drained, and flaked
2 cups cooked and cooled brown rice
½ cup frozen green peas, thawed
1 medium-sized unpeeled raw zucchini, diced
½ cup thinly sliced scallions, including green tops
6 cherry tomatoes, cut in half

DRESSING:
½ cup low-fat plain yogurt
3 tablespoons reduced-calorie mayonnaise
2 tablespoons lemon juice
2 tablespoons finely chopped fresh parsley leaves
½ teaspoon dried marjoram leaves
¼ teaspoon dried dill weed
Salt and ground black pepper to taste

In a large bowl, gently toss the salad ingredients together. In a small bowl, combine the dressing ingredients and mix well. Toss the dressing gently with the salad mixture. Refrigerate, covered, for a few hours to let the flavors mingle.

Makes 4 main-dish servings (970); about 240 calories per serving.

18

Main Dishes—Vegetarian

BAKED POTATOES WITH DILLED DAIRY TOPPING

The quantity and types of herbs in the topping may be adjusted to taste.

1 (15-ounce) container part-skim (low-fat) ricotta cheese
½ cup low-fat plain yogurt
1 garlic clove, pressed or finely minced
2 tablespoons chopped fresh parsley leaves
1 tablespoon finely chopped fresh chives or scallion greens
1 teaspoon dried dill weed OR 1 tablespoon chopped fresh
    dill weed
½ teaspoon dried basil leaves
¼ teaspoon dried marjoram leaves
Pinch of ground black pepper

TO SERVE:

4 medium-sized (about 6 ounces each) baking potatoes, such as Idaho or russet

Extra parsley sprigs or chopped fresh parsley for garnish

Put the ricotta cheese in a food processor fitted with a steel blade and process until smooth and creamy. Add the remaining ingredients except the potatoes and pulse-process 2 or 3 times —no more. If the topping is processed too much after the yogurt has been added, it will thin out.

If a food processor is not available, beat the ricotta with an electric mixer or by hand, then fold in the remaining ingredients. The topping will not be as creamy smooth as one made in a food processor.

Chill the topping, covered, for at least 1 hour (up to overnight) to let the flavors mingle.

Meanwhile, scrub the potatoes well and pierce them in several places. Bake them in a conventional oven or microwave oven until tender. To serve, cut each hot potato in half lengthwise and fluff the flesh with a fork. Top with one-fourth of the topping and garnish with the parsley. If a warm topping is preferred, the sauce may be gently heated, stirring constantly, until just warmed through.

Makes 4 main-dish servings (1080); about 270 calories per serving.

HEARTY LENTIL SOUP/STEW

This dish—which may be thought of as a very thick soup or as a bean-and-vegetable stew—is quite satisfying, and the complementary combination of lentils and brown rice provides plenty of high-quality protein.

¾ cup dry lentils, sorted and well rinsed
½ cup uncooked brown rice
2¾ cups vegetable, beef, or chicken bouillon made from cubes
  or powder
1 (16-ounce) can tomatoes, including juice, coarsely chopped
3 stalks celery, thinly sliced
2 medium-sized carrots, thinly sliced
1 large onion, finely chopped
2 tablespoons finely chopped fresh parsley leaves
1 teaspoon dried marjoram leaves
½ teaspoon dried thyme leaves
1 bay leaf, crumbled
⅛ to ¼ teaspoon ground black pepper

In a 3-quart or similar saucepan or Dutch oven, combine all the ingredients. Bring to a boil over high heat; then reduce the heat, cover the pan, and simmer, stirring occasionally, for about 45 minutes or until the lentils and rice are tender. If the soup/stew appears to be getting too dry and the rice is not yet tender, add a small amount of bouillon or water. Leftover soup/stew can be refrigerated and reheats very well (particularly in a microwave oven). It may even taste better on the second day. It can also be frozen, if desired.

Makes 4 main-dish servings (1065); about 265 calories per serving.

ZUCCHINI LASAGNE

In this recipe, zucchini is substituted for some of the noodles, adding to the taste and texture of the lasagne.

SAUCE:

1 large onion, finely chopped
3 tablespoons water
2 garlic cloves, minced
2 medium-sized carrots, grated
1 cup sliced fresh mushrooms
1 (16-ounce) can tomatoes, including juice, finely chopped
1 (6-ounce) can tomato paste
2 teaspoons ground oregano leaves
1 teaspoon ground basil leaves
⅛ teaspoon ground black pepper

FILLING:

4 medium-sized zucchini (about 2 pounds), stem ends trimmed
4 large lasagne noodles
2 cups 1% fat cottage cheese
1 tablespoon all-purpose flour
1 large egg white
4 ounces (1 cup, packed) grated part-skim mozzarella cheese
¼ cup finely grated Parmesan cheese

For the sauce, coat a large, deep skillet with nonstick cooking spray and preheat over medium-high heat. Add the onion and water and bring to a boil; reduce the heat and simmer until the onion is limp. Add the remaining sauce ingredients and simmer, uncovered, for about 15 minutes or until the sauce is thick and fragrant.

Meanwhile, thinly slice the zucchini lengthwise, then put the slices and some water into a large saucepan and steam or boil for about 3 minutes or until they are crisp-tender. Do not over-cook. Drain the slices thoroughly in a colander. Cook the lasagne noodles as directed on the package and drain well.

In a medium-sized bowl, combine the cottage cheese, flour, egg white, and half each of the mozzarella and Parmesan cheeses.

Coat a 9- by 13-inch baking dish with nonstick cooking spray, then spread a few tablespoons of the tomato sauce in the bottom. Arrange half the zucchini slices in the sauce. Evenly spread half the cottage cheese mixture on top. Spoon a third of the remaining tomato sauce over the cottage cheese. Cover with the lasagne noodles, then the remaining cottage cheese. Top with another third of the sauce and the remaining zucchini slices. Cover with the remaining tomato sauce and sprinkle the reserved grated cheeses on top.

Bake, uncovered, in a preheated 375°F for 30 minutes or until hot and bubbly.

Makes 6 main-dish servings (1680); about 280 calories per serving.

BROCCOLI FRITTATA

4 large eggs
3 large egg whites
2 tablespoons water
2 tablespoons chopped fresh parsley leaves
½ teaspoon dried basil leaves
¼ teaspoon dried thyme leaves
Dash of red hot pepper sauce
Pinch of salt
1 tablespoon reduced-calorie margarine
1 cup very small broccoli florets and peeled stem slices OR
  1 cup thinly sliced zucchini
3 tablespoons water
¼ cup thinly sliced sweet red bell pepper or canned
  pimiento
1 scallion, including green top, thinly sliced
3 ounces (¾ cup, packed), grated part-skim mozzarella
  cheese

In a medium-sized bowl, beat together the eggs, egg whites, water, herbs, hot pepper sauce, and salt. Set aside.

In a 10-inch nonstick skillet, melt the margarine over medium-high heat. Add the broccoli and sauté for 1 minute. Add the water to the skillet, cover tightly, reduce the heat, and steam for 3 minutes or until the broccoli is bright green and crisp-tender. Remove the cover, stir in the red pepper and scallion, and continue cooking, stirring constantly, for about 1 minute longer or until all the liquid has evaporated. Spread the vegetables evenly in the skillet.

Pour the egg mixture on top and let it cook undisturbed until the eggs are partially set. Lift the egg "pancake" with a spatula to allow any uncooked egg to run underneath. When the frittata is almost set, sprinkle the cheese on top. Cover the skillet and heat just until the cheese is melted. Slide the frittata onto a serving platter and cut it into three large wedges to serve.

Makes 3 main-dish servings (710); about 235 calories per serving.

19

Side Dishes and Quick Breads

EASY RATATOUILLE

1 teaspoon olive or vegetable oil
1 medium-sized onion, thinly sliced
1 garlic clove, minced
1 (16-ounce) can tomatoes, including juice, coarsely chopped
1 medium-sized eggplant, peeled and cubed
1 large green pepper, cut into squares
1 medium-sized zucchini, sliced
1 teaspoon dried basil leaves
½ teaspoon dried oregano leaves
⅛ teaspoon ground black pepper

Heat the oil in a large saucepan over medium-high heat; add the onion and cook, stirring constantly, until it is limp. If the onion begins to stick, add a few tablespoons of water and cook until most of the liquid evaporates. Add the remaining ingredients and simmer, covered, stirring occasionally, for 20 to 30 minutes or until all the vegetables are tender. Serve hot, at room temperature, or chilled.

Makes 5 side-dish servings (325); about 65 calories per serving.

SESAME BROCCOLI WITH MOCK HOLLANDAISE SAUCE

*3 medium-sized broccoli stalks, tops cut into florets and stems
    thinly peeled and sliced on the diagonal*
1 tablespoon reduced-calorie margarine
1 teaspoon flour
¼ cup hot water
1 tablespoon lemon juice
2 teaspoons butter-flavored granules
Pinch of ground black or white pepper
1 teaspoon sesame seeds (toasted, if desired)

Put the broccoli pieces into the top of a steamer over boiling water, or into a saucepan containing about 1 inch of boiling water, and steam for 6 to 8 minutes or until crisp-tender.

While the broccoli is cooking, prepare the mock hollandaise sauce. Melt the margarine in a small saucepan over medium heat and stir in the flour until well mixed. Gradually add the water, stirring constantly to break up any lumps. Add the lemon juice and butter-flavored granules. Cook, stirring constantly, until the sauce comes to a boil and the granules are completely dissolved. Simmer, stirring, 1 minute longer. Stir in the pepper.

Drain the broccoli and arrange on a serving platter. Pour the hot sauce over the broccoli. Sprinkle the sesame seeds on top.

Any extra hollandaise sauce may be reheated and used for topping other vegetables. It has about 20 calories per tablespoon.

Makes 4 side-dish servings (230); about 55 calories per serving.

FLORIDA CARROTS

3 cups thinly sliced carrots
½ cup orange juice
1 teaspoon honey
⅛ teaspoon ground ginger
Pinch of ground cinnamon
1½ teaspoons cornstarch
1 tablespoon water

In a medium-sized saucepan, combine the carrots, orange juice, honey, ginger, and cinnamon. Bring to a boil over medium-high heat; lower the heat and simmer, covered, about 10 minutes or until the carrots are just tender. Mix the cornstarch with the water and add to the carrots. Continue cooking, stirring, just until the sauce thickens.

Makes 4 side-dish servings (240); about 60 calories per serving.

BRAISED PARMESAN CELERY

½ cup beef bouillon made from cubes or powder
2 teaspoons butter-flavored granules
⅛ teaspoon dried marjoram leaves
8 stalks celery, cut on the diagonal into 2-inch-long sections
2 tablespoons grated Parmesan cheese

In a large skillet, bring the bouillon to a boil; reduce the heat to a simmer. Stir in the butter-flavored granules until dissolved and the herbs. Add the celery and simmer, covered, until tender, 20 to 25 minutes, basting occasionally. Raise the heat and quickly boil down the remaining liquid until most, but not all, has evaporated. Sprinkle the cheese over the celery, cover the skillet, and cook a few minutes longer or until the cheese has melted.

Makes 4 side-dish servings (125); about 30 calories per serving.

ACORN SQUASH STUFFED WITH APPLES

2 small acorn squash (about 1 pound each)
2 teaspoons honey
1 small apple, unpeeled, cored and finely chopped
Ground cinnamon

With a large, sharp knife, cut each squash in half lengthwise. Scoop out and discard the seeds and strings. (A grapefruit spoon is perfect for this task.) Rub ½ teaspoon honey inside the cavity of each squash half. Then fill each cavity with a one-fourth of the chopped apples. Finally, sprinkle each cavity and the cut edge of the squash with as much cinnamon as desired.

Arrange the squash halves, cut side up, in a baking dish. Add water about ¼ inch deep to the baking dish. Cover with a lid or piece of aluminum foil and bake in a preheated 375°F oven for 45 to 55 minutes or until the flesh is very tender when pierced with a fork.

To bake the stuffed squash in a microwave oven, arrange the halves in a circle in a baking dish with the narrow ends pointing toward the center of the dish. Cover tightly with a lid or heavy-duty plastic wrap. Microwave cook on high for 13 to 18 minutes, rotating the dish about every 3 minutes, or until the squash flesh is tender. Let the squash rest, covered, for about 5 minutes longer to complete the internal cooking.

Makes 4 side-dish servings (380); about 95 calories per serving.

RED CABBAGE AND APPLES

¼ cup water
1 teaspoon butter-flavored granules
1 small onion, finely chopped
1 small red cabbage (about 1 pound), cored and thinly sliced
1 large apple, unpeeled, cored and diced
1½ tablespoons apple cider vinegar
2 teaspoons dark brown sugar
Pinch of ground cloves (or to taste)
Pinch of ground black pepper (or to taste)

In a medium-sized saucepan, bring the water to a boil; add the butter-flavored granules and stir until dissolved. Reduce the heat, add the onion, and simmer until limp. Add the cabbage, cover tightly, and steam for 10 minutes. Stir in the remaining ingredients and steam for 10 minutes longer or until cabbage and apples are tender.

Makes 5 servings (295); about 60 calories per serving.

LEMONY NEW POTATOES

*1 pound new red potatoes (6 to 8 small whole ones or 4
     medium-to-large ones, halved), well scrubbed but not
     peeled*
1 tablespoon butter-flavored granules
¼ cup water
Pinch of ground black pepper
1 tablespoon lemon juice
2 tablespoons chopped pimiento
2 tablespoons chopped fresh parsley leaves

Put the potatoes in a medium-sized saucepan with water about
1 inch deep. Bring to a boil over high heat, cover, lower the
heat, and simmer for 25 to 35 minutes or until the potatoes are
tender when pierced with a fork. Drain and transfer the potatoes to a serving bowl. In the same skillet, combine the butter-
flavored granules, water, and pepper. Bring to a boil, stirring
until the granules are completely dissolved. Stir in the lemon
juice, pimiento, and parsley. Pour the sauce over the potatoes
and toss to coat them.

Makes 4 side-dish servings (380);
about 95 calories per serving.

COUNTRY COLESLAW

1 small green (white) cabbage (about 1 pound), cored and finely
*   shredded*
2 tablespoons grated onion
2 medium-sized carrots, finely shredded or grated
⅓ cup low-fat plain yogurt
2 tablespoons reduced-calorie mayonnaise
2 tablespoons apple cider vinegar
2 teaspoons sugar
¼ teaspoon powdered mustard
½ teaspoon celery seeds

In a medium-sized bowl, combine the cabbage, onion, and carrots. Add the remaining ingredients and stir well. Refrigerate,
covered, for several hours or overnight to let the flavors mingle.
Stir before serving.

Makes 6 side-dish servings (340);
about 55 calories per serving.

SWEET-AND-SOUR CABBAGE SOUP

3 cups tomato juice
1 tablespoon brown sugar
2 tablespoons cider vinegar
1 teaspoon dried basil leaves
½ teaspoon dried oregano leaves
½ teaspoon dried thyme leaves
Pinch of ground black pepper (or to taste)
1 small (about 1½ pounds) green (white) cabbage or Savoy cabbage, cored and chopped
1 cup fresh or frozen cut green beans

In a large saucepan, combine the tomato juice, sugar, vinegar, herbs, and pepper. Bring to a boil over medium-high heat, stirring occasionally. Add the cabbage and simmer, stirring occasionally, until it is limp and tender, 20 to 30 minutes. Add the green beans and continue cooking until they are just tender. Serve hot. This soup reheats well.

Makes about 6 side-dish servings (325); about 55 calories per serving.

CREAMY BROCCOLI (OR CAULIFLOWER) SOUP

2 medium-sized broccoli stalks (about 12 ounces), florets cut into small pieces and stems peeled and sliced OR about 3 cups small cauliflower florets
1 cup boiling water
1½ tablespoons reduced-calorie margarine
1½ tablespoons all-purpose flour
1¾ cups chicken bouillon made from cubes or powder
Pinch of ground black or white pepper (or to taste)
Pinch of ground nutmeg
⅓ cup instant nonfat dry milk powder
¼ cup cool water

In a medium-sized covered saucepan, over medium-high heat, steam the broccoli or cauliflower pieces in 1 cup boiling water for 5 to 8 minutes or until they are crisp-tender. In a blender or food processor, purée the broccoli or cauliflower with its cooking water. Set aside.

Rinse and dry the saucepan and put it back over medium-high heat. Melt the margarine, add the flour, and cook, stirring, for 1 minute. Slowly add the bouillon, stirring constantly, preferably with a whisk. Heat, stirring, until the mixture thickens slightly and has simmered for 2 minutes. Reduce the heat to medium; stir in the pepper, nutmeg, and puréed broccoli. Mix the milk powder with the ¼ cup water until dissolved and stir it into the soup. Cook, stirring often, until the soup is heated through.

Makes 4 side-dish servings (300); about 75 calories per serving.

EASY PUMPKIN SOUP

¼ cup water
1 tablespoon butter-flavored granules
1 small onion, very finely diced
1 stalk celery, very finely diced
2½ cups chicken or vegetable bouillon made from cubes or powder
1 (16-ounce) can pumpkin purée (NOT pumpkin pie filling)
¾ cup instant nonfat dry milk powder
½ cup cool water
¼ teaspoon ground mace or nutmeg
¼ teaspoon dried marjoram leaves
⅛ teaspoon ground allspice
⅛ teaspoon dried thyme leaves
Scant ⅛ teaspoon ground black pepper

In a medium-sized saucepan, bring the ¼ cup water to a boil over medium-high heat; stir in the butter-flavored granules until dissolved. Add the onion and celery, reduce the heat, and simmer until tender. Add the bouillon and pumpkin purée and stir until completely mixed. In a cup, dissolve the milk powder in the ½ cup cool water; stir it into the soup along with the herbs, spices, and pepper. For a very smooth, flavorful soup, purée it in batches in a blender or food processor. Before serving, reheat the soup, stirring often, until it is hot.

Makes 6 side-dish servings (400); about 65 calories per serving.

RAISIN-BRAN MUFFINS

¾ cup ready-to-eat 100% bran cereal
¾ cup cultured buttermilk
2 teaspoons vegetable oil
1 large egg white, lightly beaten
1 tablespoon light or dark molasses or brown sugar
⅓ cup all-purpose flour
¼ cup whole wheat flour
2 tablespoons raisins
1½ teaspoons baking powder
¼ teaspoon baking soda
Pinch of salt

Preheat the oven to 375°F. In a medium-sized bowl, combine the cereal and buttermilk and let rest 2 minutes. With a fork, beat in the oil, egg white, and molasses until well mixed. Add the remaining ingredients and stir just until the dry ingredients are moistened. Immediately spoon the batter into 8 nonstick spray-coated (or paper-lined) muffin cups and bake in the preheated 375°F oven for about 15 minutes or until a toothpick inserted into a muffin comes out clean. To loosen the muffins, tap the edges of the pan against the countertop. Cool the muffins slightly before serving. Extra muffins freeze well and can be quickly thawed in a microwave oven.

Makes 8 muffins (610); about 75 calories per muffin.

CORN MUFFINS

½ cup cultured buttermilk
1 large egg white
2 teaspoons sugar
1 tablespoon vegetable oil
1 tablespoon finely chopped pimiento (or fresh red pepper) (optional)
1 tablespoon finely chopped canned green chili pepper (optional)
⅔ cup stone-ground (undegerminated) cornmeal
3 tablespoons all-purpose flour
1 teaspoon baking powder
¼ teaspoon baking soda
¼ teaspoon salt

Preheat the oven to 400°F. In a small bowl, combine the buttermilk, egg white, sugar, and oil and beat with a fork until very well mixed. Add the pimiento and chili pepper (if desired), along with the cornmeal, flour, baking powder, baking soda, and salt, and stir only until the dry ingredients are completely moistened. Immediately spoon the batter into 6 nonstick spray-coated (or paper-lined) muffin cups and bake in the preheated 400°F oven for about 20 minutes or until the tops of the muffins are lightly browned. To loosen the muffins, tap the edges of the pan against the countertop. Extra muffins freeze well and can be quickly thawed in a microwave oven.

Makes 6 muffins (550); about 90 calories per muffin.

VARIATION: For Corn Sticks, bake the same batter in nonstick spray-coated corn stick pans.

WHOLE WHEAT IRISH SODA BREAD

1½ cups all-purpose or unbleached white flour
¾ cup whole wheat flour
1 tablespoon sugar
1½ teaspoons baking powder
½ teaspoon baking soda
½ teaspoon salt
2 tablespoons reduced-calorie margarine
¼ cup raisins or dried currants
1 large egg white, lightly beaten
¾ cup cultured buttermilk

Preheat the oven to 375°F. In a medium-sized bowl, mix together the flours, sugar, baking powder, baking soda, and salt. Cut in the margarine with a pastry blender or your fingertips until the mixture resembles crumbs. Stir in the raisins. Add the egg white and buttermilk and mix to form a dough. Stir several times (or knead a few times with hands) until the dough is smooth. If the dough is very moist, add a sprinkling of whole wheat flour; if it is dry and crumbly, add a few drops of buttermilk.

Coat an 8-inch round cake pan or pie plate with nonstick cooking spray and press the dough into the pan so that it fills the bottom. Use a knife to cut the traditional "X" in the top to prevent the surface from cracking.

Bake in the preheated 375°F oven for about 35 to 40 minutes

or until the top is crusty and browned and the bottom of the loaf sounds hollow when tapped. Remove the loaf from the pan and cool it on a wire rack for about 30 minutes. Serve lukewarm or at room temperature. Cut into wedges to serve.

Makes 12 wedges (1225); about 100 calories per wedge.

20

Breakfast Dishes

WAKE-UP BANANA SPLIT

1 small banana
⅓ cup 1% fat cottage cheese
¼ cup 40% bran flakes cereal
1 teaspoon chopped walnuts or hulled sunflower seeds
½ cup fresh strawberries

Peel the banana and cut it in half lengthwise. Put the halves next to each other on a plate. In a small bowl, combine the cottage cheese and bran cereal. Using an ice cream scoop or spoon, form the mixture into a ball and set it in the center of the banana halves. Sprinkle the chopped nuts or the seeds on the cottage cheese. Top with the largest, nicest strawberry and surround with remaining strawberries.

Makes 1 breakfast serving; about 205 calories per serving.

200

FRESH FRUIT WITH ORANGE–POPPY-SEED DRESSING

DRESSING:
1 cup low-fat vanilla yogurt
1 tablespoon frozen orange juice concentrate
½ teaspoon orange extract
1 teaspoon poppy seeds

FRUIT:
1 small unpeeled apple, cored and cubed
1 small unpeeled pear, cored and cubed
1 small banana, peeled and cubed
1 medium-sized orange, peeled and cubed

Combine the dressing ingredients and stir well. Store in an airtight container in the refrigerator until needed (up to 3 days) and stir before serving. Toss the fruits together. The fruit can be stored for a few days in a separate container; the juice from the orange should keep the other fruits from darkening too much.

For each serving, mix one-fourth of the fruit with one-fourth of the dressing.

Makes 4 breakfast servings (725); about 180 calories per serving.

MOCK CHEESE DANISH

1 slice whole wheat bread
¼ cup part-skim ricotta cheese
2 tablespoons unsweetened applesauce
1 large soft prune, diced
Pinch of ground cinnamon
Pinch of ground nutmeg
1 teaspoon dark brown sugar

Toast the slice of bread. Mix the cheese, applesauce, prune, cinnamon, and nutmeg and spread over the bread. Sprinkle the brown sugar on top. Heat under a broiler or in a toaster oven until hot and bubbly.

Makes 1 breakfast serving; about 195 calories per serving.

FLUFFY WHOLE WHEAT BUTTERMILK PANCAKES

½ cup cultured buttermilk
¼ teaspoon vanilla extract
2 large egg whites
¼ cup whole wheat flour
¼ cup all-purpose white flour
½ teaspoon baking soda
⅛ teaspoon ground cinnamon (optional)
⅛ teaspoon ground allspice (optional)
Pinch of cream of tartar

   TO SERVE:
2 tablespoons reduced-calorie maple-flavored syrup OR ½ cup unsweetened applesauce

In a small bowl, combine the buttermilk, vanilla extract, and 1 egg white and beat with a fork until smooth. Add the flours, baking soda, and spices (if desired). In a small bowl, beat the remaining egg white and cream of tartar until soft peaks are formed and fold it into the batter. Coat a griddle (preferably nonstick) with nonstick cooking spray and heat over medium-high heat. Spoon the batter onto the hot griddle to form pancakes. Cook until lightly browned on the bottom and several bubbles have risen to the surface; then turn and cook on the second side. Serve with syrup or applesauce.

Makes 2 breakfast servings (330); about 165 calories per serving.

DUTCH APPLE PANCAKE

½ cup skim milk
2 large egg whites
½ teaspoon vanilla extract
½ cup all-purpose flour
¼ teaspoon baking powder
1 tablespoon reduced-calorie margarine
1 medium-sized sweet, firm apple (such as Golden Delicious),
    unpeeled, cored and thinly sliced
⅛ teaspoon ground cinnamon
2 teaspoons sifted confectioner's sugar

In a small bowl, combine the milk, egg whites, and vanilla and beat with a fork until mixed. Add the flour and baking powder and mix until the batter is smooth.

In a 10-inch nonstick skillet with sloping sides, melt the margarine over medium heat; add the apple slices and evenly sprinkle the cinnamon over them. Cook the apple slices, stirring occasionally, until they are just tender, then spread them in one layer in the skillet. Pour the batter on top and tilt the skillet so the batter evenly covers the apples and fills the bottom of the skillet.

Reduce the heat to medium or medium-low and cook the pancake for about 3 minutes or until it is dry around the edges and some bubbles have formed in the top. Use a pancake turner to slide the pancake onto a large platter. Spray the skillet lightly with nonstick cooking spray. Tilt the plate to invert the pancake back into the skillet and cook about 1 minute longer on the second side or until it is cooked through. Slide it out onto a serving platter and dust with confectioner's sugar. Cut in half to serve.

If it is too difficult to slide the whole pancake out of the pan, cut it into halves or fourths and flip the piece over in the pan. The pancake might not look as attractive, but it will still taste great!

Makes 2 breakfast servings (420);
about 210 calories per serving.

COTTAGE CHEESE PANCAKES

1¼ cups 1% fat cottage cheese
1 large egg
2 large egg whites
¼ cup all-purpose flour
2 teaspoons sugar
1 teaspoon vanilla extract
1 cup unsweetened applesauce
Ground cinnamon to taste

For the smoothest pancakes, put the cottage cheese, egg, egg whites, flour, sugar, and vanilla into a food processor fitted with the steel blade. Process until the batter is creamy smooth. It will be thinner than regular pancake batter. If a food processor is not available, mix in a blender or with an electric mixer.

Coat a griddle with nonstick cooking spray and preheat it over medium heat (*no hotter*). For each pancake, spoon about 2 tablespoons of the batter onto the griddle. Cook the pancakes until they are very lightly browned on the bottom and have bubbles on top; then turn them and cook until they are very lightly browned on the second side. They do not rise very much. Serve the pancake with applesauce that is lightly sprinkled with cinnamon.

Makes 3 breakfast servings (570); about 190 calories per serving.

FRENCH TOAST WITH ORANGE-RAISIN SAUCE

1 large egg
1 large egg white
¼ cup skim milk
½ teaspoon vanilla extract
4 slices whole wheat bread
Ground cinnamon (optional)

ORANGE-RAISIN SAUCE:

¾ teaspoon cornstarch
⅓ cup orange juice
Pinch each of ground cinnamon and ginger
¼ teaspoon maple-flavor extract
2 teaspoons raisins

Put the egg and egg white in a medium-sized bowl and beat with a fork until completely combined. Beat in the milk and vanilla extract. Coat a baking sheet or shallow pan very well with nonstick cooking spray. Dip each slice of bread in the egg-milk mixture so that both sides are coated. Let any excess drip back into the bowl. Place the slices on the prepared baking sheet. If desired, lightly sprinkle the top of each slice with cinnamon. Bake in a preheated 425°F oven for about 8 minutes; then turn over the slices with a pancake turner and bake on the second side about 8 minutes longer or until lightly browned and crunchy. (An alternative method to cook the French toast is on a nonstick griddle that has been coated with nonstick cooking spray and preheated over medium-high heat.)

Meanwhile, prepare the sauce. Put the cornstarch in a small saucepan. Add a few tablespoons of the orange juice and mix until the cornstarch is dissolved. Then stir in the remaining juice, spices, maple-flavor extract, and raisins. Stir constantly over medium-high heat, until the sauce thickens slightly and just comes to a boil. To serve, spoon the warm or room-temperature sauce over the French toast.

Makes 2 breakfast servings (435);
about 215 calories per serving.

STRAWBERRY AND CHEESE CRÊPES

CRÊPES:
2 large egg whites
¼ cup instant nonfat dry milk
⅔ cup water
¼ teaspoon vanilla extract
¼ cup all-purpose white (or whole wheat) flour

FILLING:
1½ cups 1% fat cottage cheese
2 teaspoons lemon juice
1 teaspoon granulated sugar
2 cups sliced fresh strawberries
1 tablespoon sifted confectioner's sugar

Put all the crêpe ingredients in the order listed into a blender container or a food processor and process until creamy smooth, scraping down the sides of the container once during the processing. Or mix all the ingredients using an electric mixer or rotary blender. Let the batter rest for 30 minutes to 1 hour.

Preheat a 6- to 7-inch nonstick skillet with sloping sides over medium-high heat and very lightly coat it with nonstick cooking spray. Gently stir the crepe batter. Add about 2 tablespoons of the batter to the skillet and immediately tilt the skillet in all directions so that the batter forms a thin, even layer on the bottom. Cook the crêpe for 30 seconds to 1 minute or until the bottom is very lightly browned and the top is dry. Loosen the edges and turn the crêpe onto a platter. Repeat with the remaining batter, adjusting the heat if necessary. Stack the crêpes on the platter. There should be 6 to 9 crêpes.

For the filling, combine the cheese, lemon juice, and granulated sugar and mix well. Stir in half the sliced strawberries. Turn all the crêpes so the uncooked sides face upward. Evenly divide the filling among the crêpes. Roll up the crêpes and place them seam side down on a serving platter. Arrange the remaining strawberries on top. Sprinkle the confectioner's sugar over all.

Makes 3 breakfast servings (605); about 200 calories per serving.

FRUITY COOKED CEREAL

1 cup water
⅓ cup rolled oats OR ¼ cup stone-ground cornmeal OR 3 tablespoons Cream of Wheat, Cream of Rice, farina, or similar cereal
2 tablespoons instant nonfat dry milk powder
1 large pitted prune, diced
3 dried apricot halves, diced
⅛ teaspoon ground cinnamon (optional)
Pinch of salt (or to taste)
¼ cup skim milk

In a small saucepan, bring the water to a boil. Add the rolled oats, cornmeal, or dry cereal and the milk powder while stirring constantly. Stir in the prune, apricots, and cinnamon (if desired). Bring the mixture back to a boil. Reduce the heat and simmer, stirring constantly, for a few minutes or until the cereal thickens to the desired consistency. Stir in the salt. Transfer the cooked cereal to a bowl and pour the skim milk on top. Serve immediately.

Makes 1 breakfast serving; about 200 to 215 calories per serving.

21

Desserts

EASIEST-EVER RASPBERRY SHERBET

1 (10-ounce) package frozen raspberries in syrup
2 large unbeaten egg whites
1 tablespoon lemon juice
½ teaspoon vanilla extract
½ teaspoon almond extract

Partially thaw the frozen raspberries; then put the contents in a large mixing bowl and break up with a fork. Add the remaining ingredients and beat with an electric mixer at high speed for several minutes or until the mixture becomes very light and fluffy and holds stiff peaks. Spoon into 6 dessert glasses or a large bowl and freeze for several hours or until firm. (It may be stored in the freezer, covered, for up to a week.) Remove the sherbet from the freezer a few minutes before serving to give it a chance to soften slightly.

If desired, the dessert may be served as a mousse as soon as it is made; leftovers should be frozen because they will not keep well in the refrigerator. A package of frozen strawberries in syrup may be substituted for the raspberries.

Makes 6 dessert servings (310); about 50 calories per serving.

PIÑA COLADA CHIFFON SQUARES

¼ cup fine graham cracker crumbs
1 envelope unflavored gelatin
½ cup pineapple or orange juice
1 (8-ounce) can crushed pineapple in its own juice, drained and juice reserved
2 large unbeaten egg whites
½ teaspoon vanilla extract
1 teaspoon coconut extract
¼ cup sugar
4 tablespoons shredded desiccated coconut

Coat a 9-inch-square baking pan with nonstick cooking spray. Evenly distribute the graham cracker crumbs in the bottom. Soften the gelatin in ¼ cup of the juice, then heat it over very low heat until it dissolves. Remove from the heat and stir in the remaining ¼ cup juice.

Drain the pineapple and put the pineapple juice in a large mixing bowl with the egg whites and the vanilla and coconut extracts. Beat at medium speed with an electric mixer until light and foamy; slowly add the sugar and the gelatin mixture and continue beating for several minutes or until stiff peaks form. (Be patient!) Fold in the drained pineapple and 2 tablespoons of the coconut until evenly distributed. Turn the chiffon into the prepared pan. Sprinkle the remaining 2 tablespoons coconut on top (the coconut may first be lightly toasted in an oven or toaster oven, if desired, for an attractive look). Chill until firm and cool. This will take only a short while. Cut into 9 large squares to serve.

Because this dessert contains raw egg whites, it should not be stored more than 1 to 2 days.

Makes 9 dessert servings (615); about 70 calories per serving.

MICRO-BAKED STUFFED APPLE

1 small Golden Delicious or similar apple
½ teaspoon honey
1 teaspoon raisins or currants
2 tablespoons orange juice, apple juice, or cider
Ground cinnamon to taste

Core the apple through the stem end, being careful not to cut all the way through the bottom. Peel the top third of the apple only (reserve the peel) and place in a small casserole, large custard cup, or similar heatproof container. Finely chop the reserved peel and put it inside the apple cavity with the honey and raisins. Prick the peeled top of the apple with a fork. Drizzle the juice over the apple and into the cavity. Sprinkle with the cinnamon. Cover the apple with heavy-duty plastic wrap or wax paper.

Bake the apple in a microwave oven at 100 percent power for 3 to 4 minutes or until tender. About halfway through the cooking period, rotate the container once and baste the apple with the juice.

Makes 1 dessert serving; about 95 calories.

This recipe may be multiplied for additional servings; increase the microwave cooking time accordingly. Also, the apple(s) may be baked in a conventional oven at 375°F, covered, for about 45 minutes or until tender; baste periodically to keep the apples moist.

MOLDED PRUNE WHIP

3 large soft prunes, finely diced
1 envelope unflavored gelatin
1 tablespoon water
1 tablespoon sugar
⅓ cup boiling water
2 (4½-ounce) jars strained baby prunes with tapioca
½ cup instant nonfat dry milk powder
1 cup ice-cold water
2 teaspoons lemon juice
1 teaspoon vanilla extract

Chill a large mixing bowl in the freezer (or refrigerator). Lightly coat a 4-cup mold with nonstick cooking spray; then evenly distribute the diced prunes in the bottom.

In a medium-sized bowl, soften the gelatin in the 1 tablespoon water. Add the sugar and boiling water and stir until the gelatin is completely dissolved. Stir in the strained baby prunes.

Put the milk powder and ice water into the chilled bowl and beat with an electric mixer at high speed for several minutes or until light and fluffy. Add the lemon juice and vanilla and continue beating until stiff peaks are formed. Add the prune-gelatin mixture and beat until completely mixed in.

Pour into the prepared mold and chill a few hours or until the prune whip is set. Run a knife around the outside edge of the mold; then cover the mold with a platter and invert the two together while pressing downward.

Makes 6 servings (430); about 70 calories per serving.

FROZEN BANANA FUDGIES

2 medium-sized very ripe bananas, cut into chunks
⅔ cup instant nonfat dry milk powder
2½ tablespoons plain cocoa
1½ tablespoons shredded desiccated coconut

Put all the ingredients except coconut in a food processor fitted with a steel blade and process until smooth and creamy. Lightly coat an 8-inch-square pan with nonstick cooking spray; evenly spread the banana mixture in a thin, even layer. Sprinkle coconut on top. Freeze until almost firm; then cut into 64 2-inch squares (each serving = 8 small squares). Store the fudgies in a covered container in the freezer.

Makes 8 dessert servings (450); about 55 calories per serving.

PINEAPPLE SHERBET

1 (8-ounce) can crushed pineapple, including juice
1½ cups very fresh cultured buttermilk
2 tablespoons sugar OR aspartame sweetener to taste
¼ teaspoon vanilla extract OR coconut extract
¼ teaspoon orange extract

Put all the ingredients in an 8- or 9-inch-square pan (or similar pan) and mix with a spoon to combine. Freeze until firm but not solid, about 2 hours. Break the mixture up with a fork or spoon and purée in a food processor fitted with the steel blade or beat with an electric mixer until smooth and creamy. Spoon into 1 large serving dish or 5 individual dishes and freeze until firm. Before serving, allow the sherbet to soften slightly in the refrigerator or at room temperature. The sherbet may be stored for up to 1 week in the freezer, covered.

Makes 5 servings (365); about 75 calories per serving; 55 calories if aspartame sweetener is used.

MERINGUE PEARS MELBA

1 (8½-ounce) can pear halves in juice
1 large egg white
Pinch of cream of tartar
1½ tablespoons sugar
⅛ teaspoon almond extract
1 tablespoon reduced-calorie (low-sugar) raspberry or straw-
*   berry jam*

Drain the pear halves, reserving the juice in a small saucepan. Put the pear halves, cut side up, in a small baking dish. Put the egg white and cream of tartar in a mixing bowl and beat with an electric mixer until frothy. Gradually add the sugar and almond extract and continue beating until very stiff, shiny peaks form. With a spatula, swirl some of the meringue over each pear half, dividing it evenly and heaping it as necessary. Use the spatula to make peaks in the meringue. Bake the meringue-covered pears in a preheated 325°F oven for about 20 minutes or until lightly browned.

While the pears are baking, prepare the sauce. Add the jam to the juice already in the saucepan and bring to a boil over high heat. Reduce the heat and simmer, stirring often, for 5 to 8 minutes or until the jam has dissolved and the sauce has thickened slightly. When the pears are ready, spoon some of the sauce over each serving.

Makes 4 dessert servings (225); about 55 calories per serving.

STRAWBERRIES AND "CREAM"

½ cup part-skim (low-fat) ricotta cheese
2 teaspoons confectioner's sugar
½ teaspoon vanilla extract
¼ cup low-fat plain yogurt
2 cups fresh strawberries, stems and leaves removed

Put the ricotta cheese, confectioner's sugar, and vanilla extract in a food processor fitted with the steel blade or a blender. Process until very smooth. Add the yogurt and pulse-process 2 or 3 times, just until it is mixed in. Or gently fold in the yogurt by hand. (Yogurt tends to thin out when it is beaten.) Chill well. Divide the strawberries among 4 individual serving dishes and spoon the creamy topping over them.

Makes 4 dessert servings (305); about 75 calories per serving.

"ICE CREAM" BANANA POPS

More of a technique than a recipe, this dessert is surprisingly delicious and satisfying. The pops taste like rich and delectable banana ice cream; hence the name. But they won't melt and drip on the floor, as ice cream does. Part of the appeal of this dessert results from the use of wooden popsicle sticks. You can find them at most craft and toy stores.

1 medium-size just-ripe banana

Peel the banana and cut it in half crosswise. Insert 1 wooden popsicle stick into the cut end of each half, so that half the stick is inside the banana. Immediately wrap each half very tightly in plastic wrap and freeze until firm. Eat right out of the freezer.

As long as the banana pops are kept frozen and well wrapped, they will not turn brown for 2 weeks or possibly longer.

Makes 2 dessert servings (100); about 50 calories per serving.

HEIGHT AND WEIGHT

1983 Metropolitan Height and Weight Tables

WOMEN

Height Feet	Inches	Small Frame	Medium Frame	Large Frame
4	10	102–111	109–121	118–131
4	11	103–113	111–123	120–134
5	0	104–115	113–126	122–137
5	1	106–118	115–129	125–140
5	2	108–121	118–132	128–143
5	3	111–124	121–135	131–147
5	4	114–127	124–138	134–151
5	5	117–130	127–141	137–155
5	6	120–133	130–144	140–159
5	7	123–136	133–147	143–163
5	8	126–139	136–150	146–167
5	9	129–142	139–153	149–170
5	10	132–145	142–156	152–173
5	11	135–148	145–159	155–176
6	0	138–151	148–162	158–179

Weight at ages 25–59 based on lowest mortality weight in pounds according to frame (in indoor clothing weighing 3 lbs., shoes with 1″ heels).

1983 Metropolitan Height and Weight Tables

MEN

Height Feet	Inches	Small Frame	Medium Frame	Large Frame
5	2	128–134	131–141	138–150
5	3	130–136	133–143	140–153
5	4	132–138	135–145	142–156
5	5	134–140	137–148	144–160
5	6	136–142	139–151	146–164
5	7	138–145	142–154	149–168
5	8	140–148	145–157	152–172
5	9	142–148	148–160	155–176
5	10	144–154	151–163	158–180
5	11	146–157	154–166	161–184
6	0	149–160	157–170	164–188
6	1	152–164	160–174	168–192
6	2	155–168	164–178	172–197
6	3	155–168	164–178	172–197
6	4	163–176	171–187	181–207

Weight at ages 25–59 based on lowest mortality weight in pounds according to frame (in indoor clothing weighing 5 lbs., shoes with 1″ heels).

Source of basic data 1979 *Build Study*, Society of Actuaries and Association of Life Insurance Medical Directors of America,1980.

These tables are reprinted courtesy of the Metropolitan Life Insurance Company.

FOOD COMPOSITION
CONSTITUENTS OF 100 g OF EDIBLE PORTION

Name	Calories	Water, g	Protein, g	Fat, g	Ash, g	Total Carbohydrates, g	Crude Fiber, g	Total Calories	Measure	Weight in grams
				PROXIMATE COMPOSITION				AVERAGE PORTION		
DAIRY PRODUCTS										
Butter	716	15.5	.6	81	2.5	.4	0	100	1 tbsp	14
Buttermilk	36	90.5	3.5	.1	.8	5.1	0	86	1 cup	244
Cheese										
Blue mold	368	40	21.5	30.5	6.0	2.0	0	104	1 oz	28
Cheddar	398	37	25.0	32.2	3.7	2.1	0	113	1 oz (1" cube)	28
Cheddar, processed	370	40	23.2	29.9	4.9	2.0	0	105	1 oz	28
Cottage	95	76.5	19.5	.5	1.5	2.0	0	27	1 oz	28
Cream	371	51	9.0	37.0	1.0	2.0	0	106	1 oz	28
Swiss	370	39	27.5	28.0	3.8	1.7	0	105	1 oz	28
Swiss, processed	355	40	26.4	26.9	5.1	1.6	0	101	1 oz	28
Cream, light	204	72.5	2.9	20.0	.6	4.0	0	30	1 tbsp	15
Cream, whipping	330	59	2.3	35.0	.5	3.2	0	50	1 tbsp	15
Ice cream, plain	207	62.1	4.0	12.5	.8	20.6	0	167	1 slice	81
Milk, cow's										
Fluid, whole	68	87.0	3.5	3.9	.7	4.9	0	166	1 cup	244
Fluid, nonfat	36	90.5	3.5	.1	.8	5.1	0	87	1 cup	246
Evaporated, canned	138	73.7	7.0	7.9	1.5	9.9	0	346	1 cup	252
Nonfat solids, dry	362	3.5	35.6	1.0	7.9	52.0	0	28	1 tbsp	8
Malted, beverage	104	78.2	4.6	4.4	1.0	11.8	0	281	1 cup	270
Chocolate-flavored	74	83.0	3.2	2.2	.8	10.6	0	185	1 cup	250
Milk, goat's, fluid	67	87.4	3.3	4.0	.7	4.6	0	164	1 cup	244
Sherbet	123	68.1	1.5	.0	.4	30.0	—	118	½ cup	96
Whey, dried	344	6.2	12.5	1.2	7.7	72.4	0	—	—	—
FATS, OILS, AND SHORTENINGS										
Butter	716	15.5	.6	81	2.5	.4	0	100	1 tbsp	14
Fats, cooking, vegetable	884	0	0	100	0	0	0	1768	1 cup	200
Lard	902	0	0	100	0	0	0	126	1 tbsp	14
Margarine	720	15.5	.6	81	2.5	.4	0	100	1 tbsp	14
Mayonnaise	708	16	1.5	78	1.5	3.0	0	92	1 tbsp	13
Oils, salad or cooking	884	0	0	100	0	0	0	124	1 tbsp	14
Salad dressing, French	394	39.6	.6	35.5	4.0	20.3	.3	60	1 tbsp	15
Salt pork, fat	783	8.0	3.9	85	3.5	0	0	470	2 oz	60

This table (pages 217–229) is from *Human Nutrition*, third edition, by Benjamin T. Burton. Copyright © 1976 by H.J. Heinz Company. Used with permission of McGraw Hill.

FOOD COMPOSITION (continued)
CONSTITUENTS OF 100 g OF EDIBLE PORTION

		PROXIMATE COMPOSITION							AVERAGE PORTION	
Name	Cal-ories	Water, g	Pro-tein, g	Fat, g	Ash, g	Total Carbohy-drates, g	Crude Fiber, g	Total Calories	Measure	Weight in grams
FRUITS										
Berries										
Blackberries, raw	57	84.8	1.2	1.0	.5	12.5	4.2	82	1 cup	144
Blueberries, raw	61	83.4	.6	.6	.3	15.1	1.2	85	1 cup	140
Blueberries, canned, sweet	98	73	.4	.4	.2	26	1.0	245	1 cup	249
Cranberries, raw	48	87.4	.4	.7	.2	11.3	1.4	54	1 cup	113
Cranberry sauce, canned, sweet	198	48.1	.1	.3	.1	51.4	.4	550	1 cup	277
Currants, red, raw	55	84.4	1.2	.2	.6	13.6	4.0	30	½ cup	55
Gooseberries	39	88.9	.8	.2	.4	9.7	1.9	59	1 cup	150
Loganberries, raw	62	82.9	1.0	.6	.5	15.0	1.4	90	1 cup	144
Raspberries, black, raw	74	80.6	1.5	1.6	.6	15.7	6.8	100	1 cup	134
Raspberries, red, raw	57	84.1	1.2	.4	.5	13.8	4.7	70	1 cup	123
Raspberries, red, frozen	98	74.3	.7	.2	.2	24.7	2.1	84	3 oz	86
Strawberries, raw	37	89.9	.8	.5	.5	8.3	1.4	54	1 cup	149
Strawberries, frozen	95	74.8	.5	.2	.2	24.4	.6	82	3 oz	86
Citrus Fruit										
Grapefruit, raw	40	88.8	.5	.2	.4	10.1	.3	77	1 cup sections	194
Grapefruit, canned, sw.	72	79.8	.6	.2	.4	19.1	.2	181	1 cup	249
Lemons	32	89.3	.9	.6	.5	8.7	.9	20	1, 2″ diam.	100
Limes	37	86.0	.8	.1	.8	12.3	.9	19	1, 1½″ long	68
Oranges	45	87.2	.9	.2	.5	11.2	.6	70	1 med., 3″ diam.	215
Tangerines	44	87.3	.8	.3	.7	10.9	1.0	35	1 med., 2½″ diam.	114
Melons										
Cantaloupes	20	94.0	.6	.2	.6	4.6	.6	37	½, 5″ diam.	385
Honeydew	32	90.5	.5	.0	.5	8.5	.4	49	1, 2×7″ wedge	150
Watermelon	28	92.1	.5	.2	.3	6.9	.6	97	½ sl., ¾×10″	345
Tree, vine, and other fruits										
Apples, raw	58	84.1	.3	.4	.3	14.9	1.0	87	1 med. (2½″ diam.)	150
Apples, dry, uncooked	277	23	1.4	1.0	1.4	73.2	3.9	315	1 cup	114
Apricots, raw	51	85.4	1.0	.1	.6	12.9	.6	54	3	114

FOOD COMPOSITION *(continued)*
CONSTITUENTS OF 100 g OF EDIBLE PORTION

Name	Cal-ories	Water, g	Pro-tein, g	Fat, g	Ash, g	Total Carbohy-drates, g	Crude Fiber, g	Total Calories	Measure	Weight in grams
FRUITS — Continued										
Apricots,									4 med. halves,	
canned, sw.	80	77.3	.6	.1	.6	21.4	.4	97	2 tbsp	122
Apricots, dry	262	24	5.2	.4	3.5	66.9	3.2	280	40 halves	150
Avocado	245	65.4	1.7	26.4	1.4	5.1	1.8	280	½, 3½ × 3¼"	114
Bananas	88	74.8	1.2	.2	.8	23	.6	132	1 med., 6 × 1½"	150
Cherries, all,										
raw	61	83.0	1.1	.5	.6	14.8	.3	94	1 cup pitted	154
Cherries, red,										
sour, canned	48	86.6	.8	.3	.4	11.9	.1	122	1 cup pitted	254
Dates, dried	284	20	2.2	.6	1.8	75.4	2.4	505	1 cup pitted	177
Figs, canned,										
sw.	113	68.5	.8	.3	.4	30.0	.9	130	3, 2 tbsp syrup	115
Figs, dried	270	24	4.0	1.2	2.4	68.4	5.8	57	1 large, 1 × 2"	21
Grapes, raw										
American										
(slip skin)	70	81.9	1.4	1.4	.4	14.9	.5	84	1 cup	153
European										
(adherent										
skin)	66	81.6	.8	.4	.5	16.7	.5	102	1 cup, 40 grapes	160
Guavas, raw	70	80.6	1.0	.6	.7	17.1	5.5	49	1 small	80
Papaya, raw	43	88.3	.6	.1	—	10.0	—	73	1, 2½ × 7" wedge	170
Peaches,									1 med., 2½ × 2"	
raw	46	86.9	.5	.1	.5	12.0	.6	45	diam.	114
Peaches,										
canned, sw.	68	80.9	.4	.1	.4	18.2	.4	175	1 cup	258
Peaches, frozen,										
sw.	88	76.3	.5	.1	.8	22.8	.4	99	4 oz	112
Peaches, dry,										
uncooked	265	24	3.0	.6	3.0	69.4	3.5	424	1 cup	160
Pears, raw	63	82.7	.7	.4	.4	15.8	1.4	95	1, 3 × 2½" diam.	182
Pears, canned,									2 halves, 2 tbsp	
sw.	68	81.1	.2	.1	.2	18.4	.8	80	syrup	117
Plums, raw	50	85.7	.7	.2	.5	12.9	.5	30	1, 2" diam.	60
Plums, canned,										
sw.	76	78.6	.4	.1	.5	20.4	.3	186	1 cup	256
Prunes, dry	268	24	2.3	.6	2.1	71.0	1.6	94	4 large	40
Raisins, dry	268	24	2.3	.5	2.0	71.2	—	430	1 cup	160
Rhubarb,										
frozen	74	80.2	.6	.2	.6	19.2	.9	202	1 cup	273
FRUIT JUICES AND OTHER FRUIT PRODUCTS										
Apple juice, frozen										
or canned	50	85.9	.1	0	.3	13.8	—	124	1 cup	249
Apple sauce,										
frozen or										
canned, sw.	72	79.8	.2	.1	.2	19.7	.6	185	1 cup	254
Apricot nectar	52	86.1	.3	.1	.5	12.4	.2	170	1 cup	254

FOOD COMPOSITION (continued)
CONSTITUENTS OF 100 g OF EDIBLE PORTION

Name	Calories	Water, g	Protein, g	Fat, g	Ash, g	Total Carbohydrates, g	Crude Fiber, g	Total Calories	Measure	Weight in grams
						PROXIMATE COMPOSITION			AVERAGE PORTION	

FRUIT JUICES AND OTHER FRUIT PRODUCTS—Continued

Name	Calories	Water, g	Protein, g	Fat, g	Ash, g	Total Carbohydrates, g	Crude Fiber, g	Total Calories	Measure	Weight in grams
Fruit cocktail, canned, sweet	70	80.6	.4	.2	.3	18.6	.4	180	1 cup	257
Grape juice, canned, sw.	67	81	.4	0	.4	18.2	—	120	6 oz	180
Grapefruit juice, canned, sweet	52	85.3	.5	.1	.4	13.7	.1	131	1 cup	251
Lemon juice, canned	24	91.4	.4	.2	.3	7.7	0	4	1 tbsp	15
Lime juice, fresh	24	91.0	.4	0	.3	8.3	0	57	1 cup	246
Olives, green	132	75.2	1.5	13.5	5.8	4.0	1.2	72	10 "mammoth"	65
Olives, ripe, Mission	191	71.8	1.8	21.0	2.8	2.6	1.5	106	10 "mammoth"	65
Orange juice, fresh	44	87.5	.8	.2	.4	11.0	.1	108	1 cup	246
Orange juice, canned	44	87.5	.8	.2	.4	11.1	.1	135	1 cup	251
Orange and grapefruit juice, canned, sw.	52	85.1	.5	.1	.4	13.9	.1	132	1 cup	251
Pineapple juice, canned	49	86.2	.3	.1	.4	13.0	.1	121	1 cup	249
Prune juice, canned	71	80	.4	0	.3	19.3	—	170	1 cup	240
Tangerine juice, canned	39	89.2	.9	.3	.4	9.2	—	95	1 cup	246
Tomato juice, canned	21	93.5	1.0	.2	1.0	4.3	.2	50	1 cup	242

GRAINS AND GRAIN PRODUCTS
Breakfast cereals

Name	Calories	Water, g	Protein, g	Fat, g	Ash, g	Total Carbohydrates, g	Crude Fiber, g	Total Calories	Measure	Weight in grams
Bran flakes	292	3.6	10.8	1.9	4.9	78.8	3.9	117	1 cup	40
Corn flakes*	385	3.6	8.1	.4	2.9	85.0	.6	96	1 cup	25
Farina, cooked	44	89.2	1.3	.1	.3	9.1	0	105	1 cup	238
Oat breakfast cereal*	396	4.0	14.5	7.0	4.3	70.2	2.0	100	1 cup	25
Oatmeal, cooked	63	84.8	2.3	1.2	.7	11.0	.2	150	1 cup	238
Puffed rice*	392	3.5	5.9	.6	2.3	87.7	.5	55	1 cup	14
Puffed wheat*	355	3.8	10.8	1.6	3.6	80.2	1.7	43	1 cup	12
Rice flakes*	392	3.5	5.9	.6	2.3	87.7	.5	117	1 cup	30
Wheat flakes*	355	3.8	10.8	1.6	3.6	80.2	1.7	125	1 cup	35
Wheat, whole meal*	344	8.2	12.7	1.7	2.1	75.3	2.2	103	¼ cup	30

*Enriched, fortified, or restored to legal standard when one exists.

FOOD COMPOSITION *(continued)*
CONSTITUENTS OF 100 g OF EDIBLE PORTION

	PROXIMATE COMPOSITION							AVERAGE PORTION		
Name	Cal-ories	Water, g	Pro-tein, g	Fat, g	Ash, g	Total Carbohy-drates, g	Crude Fiber, g	Total Calories	Measure	Weight in grams
FLOURS, MEALS, AND OTHER FARINACEOUS MATERIALS										
Barley, pearled, light	349	11.1	8.2	1.0	.9	78.8	.5	710	1 cup	204
Buckwheat flour, light	348	12	6.4	1.2	.9	79.5	.5	342	1 cup	98
Corn grits*, cooked	51	87.1	1.2	.1	.6	11.0	.1	122	1 cup	242
Cornmeal, whole	362	12	9.0	3.4	1.1	74.5	1.0	459	1 cup	127
Cornmeal, degermed*	363	12	7.9	1.2	.5	78.4	.6	527	1 cup	145
Farina*	370	10.5	10.9	.8	.4	77.4	.4	625	1 cup	169
Flour, rye, dark	318	11	16.3	2.6	2.0	68.1	2.4	285	1 cup	80
Flour, wheat, 80% extn.	365	12	12.0	1.3	.7	74.1	.5	400	1 cup, stirred	110
Flour, wheat, self-rising*	350	12	9.2	1.0	4.0	73.8	.4	384	1 cup, stirred	110
Flour, wheat, all-purpose*	364	12	10.5	1.0	.4	76.1	.3	400	1 cup, stirred	110
Flour, wheat, cake	364	12	7.5	.8	.3	79.4	.2	364	1 cup, stirred	100
Rice, brown	360	12	7.5	1.7	1.1	77.7	.6	748	1 cup	208
Rice, converted	362	12	7.6	.3	.4	79.4	.2	677	1 cup	187
Rice, white	362	12.3	7.6	.3	.4	79.4	.2	692	1 cup	191
Soybean flour, defatted	228	11.0	44.7	1.1	5.5	37.7	2.3			
Starch, pure	362	12	.5	.2	.3	87	.1	29	1 tbsp	8
Tapioca, dry	360	12.6	.6	.2	.2	86.4	.1	547	1 cup	152
Wheat germ	361	11.0	25.2	10.0	4.3	49.5	2.5	246	1 cup	68
Wild rice	364	8.5	14.1	.7	1.4	75.3	1.0	593	1 cup	163
BAKED AND COOKED PRODUCTS										
Breads										
Boston brown*	219	44.5	4.8	2.1	2.6	46.0	.3	105	1, ¾" slice	48
Cracked wheat*	259	36.0	8.5	2.2	1.9	51.4	.5	60	1, ½" slice	23
French or Vienna*	270	35.5	8.1	2.7	1.7	52.0	.2	1225	1 lb	453
Raisin	284	30.2	7.1	3.1	1.8	57.8	.2	65	1, ½" slice	23
Rye (⅓ rye flour)	244	35.3	9.1	1.2	2.0	52.4	.4	57	1, ½" slice	23
White, 4% nonfat milk solids*	275	34.7	8.5	3.2	1.8	51.8	.2	63	1, ½" slice	23
Whole wheat	240	36.6	9.3	2.6	2.5	49.0	1.5	55	1, ½" slice	23
Bread crumbs, dry	385	8.5	11.9	4.5	2.6	72.5	.2	339	1 cup	88
Cakes										
Angel food	270	31.6	8.4	.3	1.0	58.7	0	110	2" sec. of 8" cake	41
Foundation	350	25.1	5.9	11.7	1.4	55.9	.1	230	1 sq., 3 × 2 × 1¾"	66
Fruit, dark	354	22.9	5.2	13.8	2.2	55.9	1.2	106	2 × 2 × ½"	30
Plain	327	26.8	6.4	8.2	1.6	57.0	.1	161	1, 2¾" cupcake	50

*Enriched, fortified, or restored to legal standard when one exists.

FOOD COMPOSITION (continued)
CONSTITUENTS OF 100 g OF EDIBLE PORTION

Name		PROXIMATE COMPOSITION							AVERAGE PORTION	
	Cal-ories	Water, g	Pro-tein, g	Fat, g	Ash, g	Total Carbohy-drates, g	Crude Fiber, g	Total Calories	Measure	Weight in grams
BAKED AND COOKED PRODUCTS—Continued										
Sponge	291	31.8	7.9	5.0	.9	54.4		117	2″ sec. of 8″ cake	40
Corn bread*	219	49.2	6.7	4.7	2.8	36.6	.2	103	1, 2¾″ muffin	48
Crackers, graham	393	5.5	8.0	10.0	2.2	74.3	.8	55	2 medium	14
Crackers, saltines	431	4.6	9.2	11.8	3.3	71.1	.4	34	2, 2″ square	8
Custard, baked	114	77.3	5.3	5.4	.8	11.2	0	283	1 custard cup	248
Doughnuts	425	18.7	6.6	21.0	1.0	52.7	.2	136	1	32
Fig bars	350	13.8	4.2	4.8	1.4	75.8	1.7	87	1 large bar	25
Gingerbread	327	30.4	3.9	12.0	2.1	51.6	.1	180	1, 2″ cube	55
Macaroni,* dry	377	8.6	12.8	1.4	.7	76.5	.4	463	1 cup dry	123
Macaroni and cheese, cooked	211	58.1	8.1	11.0	3.1	19.7	.1	464	1 cup	220
Muffins*	280	37.4	8.0	8.4	2.2	42.1	.1	135	1, 2¾″ muffin	48
Noodles (egg), cooked	67	83.8	2.2	.6	.6	12.8	.1	107	1 cup	60
Pancakes, wheat*	218	55.4	6.8	9.2	2.0	26.6	.1	60	1, 4″ diam.	27
Pancakes, buckwheat	176	62.0	6.1	8.4	2.6	20.9	.5	48	1, 4″ diam.	27
Pies										
Apple	246	47.8	2.1	9.5	1.1	39.5	.7	330	4″ sec. of 9″ pie	220
Mince	252	43.0	2.5	6.9	2.0	45.6	.5	340	4″ sec. of 9″ pie	135
Pumpkin	202	58.9	4.2	9.6	1.5	25.8	.6	265	4″ sec. of 9″ pie	131
Pretzels	369	8.0	8.8	3.2	5.5	74.5	.3	18	5 small sticks	5
Rolls, plain*	309	28.5	9.0	5.5	1.9	55.1	.2	120	1 (1/12 lb)	39
Rolls, sweet	323	28.4	8.5	7.8	1.5	53.8	.2	178	1	55
Rye wafers	324	6.5	12.4	1.2	4.6	75.3	2.1	43	2	13
Spaghetti,* cooked	149	60.6	5.1	.6	3.5	30.2	.2	220	1 cup	148
Waffles*	287	40	9.3	10.6	2.3	37.8	.1	216	1, 4½ × 5⅝ × ½″	75
NUTS AND NUT PRODUCTS										
Almonds, dry	597	4.7	18.6	54.1	3.0	19.6	2.7	850	1 cup	140
Brazil nuts, shelled	646	5.3	14.4	65.9	3.4	11.0	2.1	905	1 cup	140
Cashews, roasted	578	3.6	18.5	48.2	2.7	27.0	1.3	810	1 cup	140
Chestnuts, fresh	191	53.2	2.8	1.5	1.0	41.5	1.1	95	20	250
Coconut, dry, sw.	556	3.3	3.6	39.1	.8	53.2	4.1	344	1 cup shreds	62
Peanuts, roasted	559	2.6	26.9	44.2	2.7	23.6	2.4	805	1 cup	144
Peanut butter	576	1.7	26.1	47.8	3.4	21.0	2.0	92	1 tbsp	16
Pecans, raw	696	3.0	9.4	73.0	1.6	13.0	2.2	752	1 cup of halves	108
Walnuts, Eng., raw	654	3.3	15.0	64.4	1.7	15.6	2.1	654	1 cup of halves	100

*Enriched, fortified, or restored to legal standard when one exists.

FOOD COMPOSITION *(continued)*
CONSTITUENTS OF 100 g OF EDIBLE PORTION

Name	Calories	Water, g	Protein, g	Fat, g	Ash, g	Total Carbohydrates, g	Crude Fiber, g	Total Calories	Measure	Weight in grams
			PROXIMATE COMPOSITION					AVERAGE PORTION		
MEAT										
Beef										
Chuck, cooked	309	51	26	22	.7	0	0	265	3 oz	86
Hamburger, cooked	364	47	22	30	1.1	0	0	316	3 oz	86
Porterhouse, cooked	342	49	23	27	1.1	0	0	293	3 oz	86
Rib roast, cooked	319	51	24	24	1.2	0	0	266	3 oz	86
Round, cooked	233	59	27	13	1.3	0	0	197	3 oz	86
Corned beef, canned	216	59.3	25.3	12	3.4	0	0	180	3 oz	86
Corned beef hash, canned	141	70.4	13.7	6.1	2.6	7.2	.2	120	3 oz	86
Dried or chipped beef	203	47.7	34.3	6.3	11.6	0	0	115	2 oz	56
Roast beef, canned	224	60	25	13	2	0	0	189	3 oz	86
Lamb										
Med. fat, raw	317	55.8	15.7	27.7	.8	0	0	273	3 oz	86
Rib chop, raw	356	51.9	14.9	32.4	.8	0	0	409	4 oz	115
Rib chop, cooked	418	40	24	35	1.2	0	0	480	4 oz	115
Leg roast, raw	235	63.7	18.0	17.5	.9	0	0	202	3 oz	86
Leg roast, cooked	274	56	24	19	1.1	0	0	314	3 oz	86
Pork										
Bacon, fried	607	13	25	55	6	1	0	97	2 slices	16
Bacon, Canadian, raw	231	56	22.1	15	6.2	.3	0	262	4 oz	115
Ham, fresh, raw	344	53	15.2	31	.8	0	0	296	3 oz	86
Ham, cured, cooked	397	39	23	33	5.4	.4	0	340	3 oz	86
Pork luncheon meat, canned	289	55.2	14.9	24.3	4.1	1.5	.2	165	2 oz	57
Veal										
Veal, med. fat	190	68	19.1	12	1.0	0	0	219	4 oz	115
Veal cutlet, cooked	219	60	28	11	1.4	0	0	184	3 oz	86
Stew meat, cooked	296	53	25	21	.8	0	0	252	3 oz	86
VARIETY MEATS AND MIXTURES										
Brains	125	78.9	10.4	8.6	1.4	.8	0	106	3 oz	86
Chili con carne	200	66.9	10.3	14.8	2.2	5.8	.2	170	⅓ cup	85
Heart, beef, raw	108	77.6	16.9	3.7	1.1	.7	0	92	3 oz	86
Kidneys, beef, raw	141	74.9	15.0	8.1	1.1	.9	0	120	3 oz	86

FOOD COMPOSITION (continued)
CONSTITUENTS OF 100 g OF EDIBLE PORTION

	PROXIMATE COMPOSITION						AVERAGE PORTION		
Name	Cal-ories	Water, g	Pro-tein, g	Fat, g	Ash, g	Total Carbohy-drates, g	Crude Fiber, g	Total Calories	Measure	Weight in grams

Name	Cal-ories	Water, g	Pro-tein, g	Fat, g	Ash, g	Carbohy-drates, g	Crude Fiber, g	Total Calories	Measure	Weight in grams
VARIETY MEATS AND MIXTURES—Continued										
Liver, beef, raw	136	69.7	19.7	3.2	1.4	6.0	0	117	3 oz	86
Liver, beef, fried	208	57.2	23.6	7.7	1.8	9.7	0	118	2 oz	57
Liver, calf, raw	141	70.8	19.0	4.9	1.3	4.0	0	121	3 oz	86
Liver, pork, raw	134	72.3	19.7	4.8	1.5	1.7	0	115	3 oz	86
Sausage, bologna	221	62.4	14.8	15.9	3.3	3.6	—	117	2 slices, ⅛ × 4″	211
Sausage, frankfurter, cooked	248	62	14	20	2	2	—	124	1, 7 × ¾″	51
Sausage, liverwurst	263	59.0	16.7	20.6	2.2	1.5	—	150	2 oz	57
Sausage, pork, raw	450	41.9	10.8	44.8	2.1	0	0	158	2, 3½″ long	35
Sweetbreads, cooked	178	67.2	22.7	9.1	—	0	0	204	4 oz	115
Tongue, beef	207	68	16.4	15	.9	.4	0	235	4 oz	115
FISH AND SEAFOODS										
Bluefish, baked	155	69.2	27.4	4.2	1.9	0	0	178	4 oz	115
Caviar, sturgeon	243	57.0	26.9	15.0	—	—	0	208	3 oz	86
Clams, raw	81	80.3	12.8	1.4	2.1	3.4	0	92	4 oz	115
Cod, raw	74	82.6	16.5	4	1.2	0	0	85	4 oz	115
Cod, dried	375	12.3	81.8	2.8	7.0	0	0	106	1 oz	28
Crabs, canned or cooked	104	77.2	16.9	2.9	1.7	1.3	0	90	3 oz	86
Flounder, raw	68	82.7	14.9	.5	1.3	0	0	78	4 oz	115
Frog legs, raw	73	81.9	16.4	.3	1.1	0	0	82	4 oz	115
Haddock, cooked	158	66.9	18.7	5.5	1.9	7.0	0	158	1 fillet, 4 × 3 × ½″	100
Halibut, raw	126	75.4	18.6	5.2	1.0	0	0	145	4 oz	115
Halibut, cooked	182	64.2	26.2	7.8	1.9	0	0	230	1 fillet, 4 × 3 × ½″	126
Herring, raw	191	67.2	18.3	12.5	2.7	0	0	191	1 small	100
Herring, kippered	211	61.0	22.2	12.9	4.0	0	0	211	1 small	100
Lobster, raw	88	79.2	16.2	1.9	2.2	.5	0	88	½ average	100
Lobster, canned	92	77.2	18.4	1.3	2.7	.4	0	78	3 oz	86
Mackerel, canned	182	66.0	19.3	11.1	3.2	0	0	155	3 oz	86
Oysters, raw	84	80.5	9.8	2.1	2.0	5.6	0	200	13–19 med., 1 cup	238
Oyster stew	91	82.6	5.3	5.4	1.4	5.3	0	244	1 cup, 6–8 oysters	240
Salmon, raw	223	63.4	17.4	16.5	1.0	0	0	192	3 oz	86
Salmon, canned	203	64.7	19.7	13.2	2.4	0	0	120	3 oz	86
Sardines, canned	214	57.4	25.7	11.0	4.7	1.2	0	182	3 oz, drained	86
Pilchards, canned	200	65.2	17.7	13.5	2.9	.7	0	171	3 oz	86
Scallops, raw	78	80.3	14.8	.1	1.4	3.4	0	90	4 oz	115
Shad, raw	168	70.2	18.7	9.8	1.4	0	0	191	4 oz	115
Shrimp, canned	127	66.2	26.8	1.4	5.8	—	0	110	3 oz	86
Swordfish, cooked	178	64.8	27.4	6.8	1.7	0	0	223	1 steak, 3 × 3 × ½″	125
Tuna fish, canned	198	60.0	29.0	8.2	2.7	0	0	170	3 oz, drained solids	86

FOOD COMPOSITION *(continued)*
CONSTITUENTS OF 100 g OF EDIBLE PORTION

Name	Cal-ories	Water, g	Pro-tein, g	Fat, g	Ash, g	Total Carbohy-drates, g	Crude Fiber, g	Total Calories	Measure	Weight in grams
PROXIMATE COMPOSITION								**AVERAGE PORTION**		
POULTRY AND EGGS										
Chicken, fryers, raw	112	74.5	20.5	2.7	1.1	0	0	210	1 breast	224
Chicken, roasters, raw	200	66.0	20.2	12.6	1.0	0	0	227	4 oz	115
Chicken, canned	199	61.9	29.8	8.0	2.4	0	0	169	3 oz	86
Chicken liver	141	69.6	22.1	4.0	1.7	2.6	0	106	2 med. livers	75
Duck	322	54.3	16.1	28.6	1.0	0	—	370	4 oz	115
Goose	366	49.7	15.9	33.6	.9	0	0	420	4 oz	115
Turkey	268	58.3	20.1	20.2	1.0	0	0	304	4 oz	115
Eggs, raw										
White	50	87.8	10.8	0	.6	.8	0	15	1 white	31
Yolk	361	49.4	16.3	31.9	1.7	.7	0	61	1 yolk	17
Whole	162	74.0	12.8	11.5	1.0	.7	0	77	1 medium egg	54
Eggs, dried										
White	398	3	85.9	0	4.8	6.3	0	223	1 cup whites	56
Yolk	693	3	31.2	61.2	3.3	1.3	0	666	1 cup yolks	96
Whole	592	5	46.8	42.0	3.6	2.5	0	640	1 cup	108
SUGARS AND SWEETS										
Candied peel										
Citron	314	18.0	.2	.3	1.3	80.2	1.4	89	1 oz	28
Ginger root	340	12	.3	.2	.4	87.1	.7	85	1 small piece	25
Lemon, orange, or grapefruit	316	17.4	.4	.3	1.3	80.6	2.3	32	1 small piece	10
Butterscotch	410	5.0	0	8.9	.5	85.6	0	20	¾″ sq. × ⅜″	5
Caramels	415	7.0	2.9	11.6	1	77.5	0	42	⅞″ sq. × ½″	10
Chocolate, sweetened, milk	503	1.1	6	33.5	1.7	55.7	.5	30	¾ × 1½ × ¼″	6
Chocolate, with almonds	532	.6	8	38.6	1.8	50.0	.6	32	¾ × 1½ × ¼″	6
Chocolate creams	394	9	4	14	1	72	—	55	1¼″ diam. × ¾″	14
Fondant	352	8	0	0	1	91	0	28	1″ sq. × ⅝″	8
Fudge, plain	411	5	1.7	11.3	.7	81.3	.3	185	2″ sq. × ⅝″	45
Hard candy	383	1	0	0	0	99	0	31	3, ¾″ diam.	8
Marshmallows	325	15	3	0	1	81	—	98	5, 1¼″ diam.	30
Peanut brittle	441	2	8.3	15.5	1.3	72.8	.8	66	1½ × 3″	15
Chocolate, bitter	501	2.3	5.5	52.9	3.2	29.2	2.6	30	¾ × 1½ × ¼″	6
Chocolate, plain, sw.	471	1.4	2	29.8	1.4	62.7	1.4	28	¾ × 1½ × ¼″	6
Chocolate syrup	209	39.0	1.2	1.1	.6	56.6	.6	40	1 tbsp	19
Cocoa, breakfast	293	3.9	8	23.8	5.0	48.9	4.6	15	2 tsp	5
Cocoa beverage, all milk	95	79.0	3.8	4.6	.9	10.9	.1	236	1 cup	250
Honey	294	20	.3	0	.2	79.5	—	62	1 tbsp	21
Jams, marmalades, etc.	278	28	.5	.3	.4	70.8	.6	55	1 tbsp	20
Jellies	252	34.5	.2	0	.3	65.0	0	50	1 tbsp	20

FOOD COMPOSITION *(continued)*
CONSTITUENTS OF 100 g OF EDIBLE PORTION

Name	\n PROXIMATE COMPOSITION						AVERAGE PORTION		
	Cal-ories	Water, g	Pro-tein, g	Fat, g	Ash, g	Total Carbohy-drates, g	Crude Fiber, g	Total Calories	Measure	Weight in grams
SUGARS AND SWEETS—Continued										
Molasses, cane, light	252	24	—	—	6.3	65	—	50	1 tbsp	20
Molasses, cane, blackstrap	213	24	—	—	.5	55	—	43	1 tbsp	20
Syrup, table blends	286	25	0	0	.6	74	—	57	1 tbsp	20
Sugars, cane or beet	385	.5	0	0	0	99.5	0	48	1 tbsp	12
Sugar, brown	370	3	0	0	1.2	95.5	—	51	1 tbsp	14
Corn sugar	348	7.5	—	—	.3	90	—	45	1 tbsp	13
Maple sugar	348	7.5	—	—	.9	90	—	104	Piece 1¾ × 1¼ × ½"	30
ROOT AND TUBER VEGETABLES										
Beets, red, raw	42	87.6	1.6	.1	1.1	9.6	.9	56	1 cup, diced	134
Beets, cooked	41	88.3	1.0	.1	.8	9.8	.8	68	1 cup, cooked, diced	165
Beets, canned	34	90.3	.9	.1	.8	7.9	.5	82	Canned, 1 cup	246
Carrots, raw	42	88.2	1.2	.3	1.0	9.3	1.1	45	Grated, 1 cup	110
Carrots, canned	30	91.5	.6	.5	1.0	6.4	.8	44	Diced, 1 cup	145
Parsnips, raw	78	78.6	1.5	.5	1.2	18.2	2.2	94	⅔ cup, diced	120
Parsnips, cooked	60	83.5	1.0	.5	1.1	13.9	2.1	94	Diced, 1 cup	155
Potatoes, sweet, raw	123	68.5	1.8	.7	1.1	27.9	1.0	185	1, 6 × 1¾"	150
Potatoes, sweet, boiled	123	68.5	1.8	.7	1.1	27.9	1.0	252	1, 5 × 2.5"	205
Potatoes, sweet, candied	179	57.4	1.5	3.6	1.3	36.2	.8	270	1, 6 × 1¾", candied	150
Potatoes, white, raw	83	77.8	2.0	.1	1.0	19.1	.4	83	1 med., 2½" diam.	100
Potatoes, white, baked	98	73.8	2.4	.1	1.2	22.5	.5	97	1 med., 2½" diam.	100
Potatoes, white, boiled	83	77.8	2.0	.1	1.0	19.1	.4	120	1 med.	142
Radishes, raw	20	93.6	1.2	.1	1.0	4.2	.7	4	4 small	40
Rutabagas, raw	38	89.1	1.1	.1	.8	8.9	1.3	45	Diced, ¾ cup	120
Rutabagas, cooked	32	90.8	.8	.1	.8	7.5	1.4	50	Cooked, diced, 1 cup	155
Turnips, raw	32	90.9	1.1	.2	.7	7.1	1.1	43	1 cup, diced	134
Turnips, cooked	27	92.3	.8	.2	.7	6.0	1.2	42	1 cup, diced	155
LEAF AND STEM VEGETABLES										
Asparagus, raw	21	93.0	2.2	.2	.7	3.9	.7	16	6, 6" stalks	75
Asparagus, cooked	20	92.5	2.4	.2	1.3	3.6	.8	36	1 cup cut spears	175
Asparagus, canned	18	93.6	1.9	.3	1.3	2.9	.5	22	6 med. spears	126
Beet greens, raw	27	90.4	2.0	.3	1.7	5.6	1.4	27	1 cup	100

FOOD COMPOSITION *(continued)*
CONSTITUENTS OF 100 g OF EDIBLE PORTION

Name		PROXIMATE COMPOSITION						AVERAGE PORTION		
	Cal-ories	Water, g	Pro-tein, g	Fat, g	Ash, g	Total Carbohy-drates, g	Crude Fiber, g	Total Calories	Measure	Weight in grams
LEAF AND STEM VEGETABLES—Continued										
Beet greens, cooked	27	90.4	2.0	.3	1.7	5.6	1.4	39	1 cup	145
Brussels sprouts, raw	47	84.9	4.4	.5	1.3	8.9	1.3	47	1 cup	100
Brussels sprouts, cooked	47	84.9	4.4	.5	1.3	8.9	1.3	60	1 cup, cooked	130
Brussels sprouts, frozen	36	88.4	3.3	.2	.9	7.3	1.3	36	1 cup	100
Cabbage, raw	24	92.4	1.4	.2	.8	5.3	1.0	24	Shredded, 1 cup	100
Cabbage, cooked	24	92.4	1.4	.2	.8	5.3	1.0	40	Cooked, diced, 1 cup	170
Celery, raw	18	93.7	1.3	.2	1.1	3.7	.7	18	Raw, diced, 1 cup	100
Chard, leaves, raw	27	91	2.6	.4	1.2	4.8	.8	27	Leaves, 1½ cups	100
Chard, leaves and stalks, cooked	21	91.8	1.4	.2	2.2	4.4	.9	30	1 cup	145
Chicory, French endive	21	94.2	1.6	.3	1.0	2.9	.8	3	¼ sm. head	15
Chives	52	86.0	3.8	.6	1.8	7.8	2.0	4	1 tbsp. chopped	7
Dandelion greens, cooked	44	85.8	2.7	.7	2.0	8.8	1.8	80	1 cup greens, cooked	180
Endive, raw	20	93.3	1.6	.2	.9	4.0	.8	90	1 lb, raw	460
Kale, raw	40	86.6	3.9	.6	1.7	7.2	1.2	70	1¾ cup	175
Kale, frozen	32	89.8	3.2	.5	.9	5.6	.9	56	1¾ cup	175
Kohlrabi, raw	30	90.1	2.1	.1	1.0	6.7	1.1	41	1 cup	138
Lettuce, headed	15	94.8	1.2	.2	.9	2.9	.6	7	2 lg. or 4 sm. leaves	50
Mustard greens, cooked	22	92.2	2.3	.3	1.2	4.0	.8	31	1 cup greens	140
Onions, mature, raw	45	87.5	1.4	.2	.6	10.3	.1	50	1, 2½″ diam.	110
Onions, mature, cooked	38	89.5	1.0	.2	.6	8.7	.8	79	1 cup	210
Onions, young green	45	87.6	1.0	.2	.6	10.6	1.8	23	6 small, less tops	50
Parsley	50	83.9	3.7	1.0	2.4	9.0	1.8	1	1 tbsp	3.5
Sauerkraut, canned	22	91.2	1.4	.3	2.7	4.4	.9	32	Canned, drained, 1 cup	150
Spinach, raw	20	92.7	2.3	.3	1.5	3.2	.6	22	Raw, 4 oz	115
Spinach, cooked	26	90.8	3.1	.6	1.9	3.6	1.0	46	Cooked, 1 cup	80
Spinach, canned	20	92.3	2.3	.4	1.8	3.0	.7	45	Canned, 1 cup	232
Turnip greens, raw	30	89.5	2.9	.4	1.8	5.4	1.2	15	Raw, ½ cup	50
Turnip greens, cooked	30	89.5	2.9	.4	1.8	5.4	1.2	43	Cooked, 1 cup	145
Watercress	18	93.6	1.7	.3	1.1	3.3	.5	5	½ cup	20

FOOD COMPOSITION (continued)
CONSTITUENTS OF 100 g OF EDIBLE PORTION

Name	PROXIMATE COMPOSITION							AVERAGE PORTION		
	Cal-ories	Water, g	Pro-tein, g	Fat, g	Ash, g	Total Carbohy-drates, g	Crude Fiber, g	Total Calories	Measure	Weight in grams
FLOWER, FRUIT, AND SEED VEGETABLES										
Artichoke	63	83.7	2.9	.4	1.1	11.9	3.2	33	1, 3″ diam.	50
Beans										
Red kidney, raw, dry	336	12.2	23.1	1.7	3.6	59.4	3.5	638	1 cup	190
Red kidney, canned or cooked	90	76.0	5.7	.4	1.5	16.4	.9	230	1 cup	255
Others, raw, dry	338	11.5	21.4	1.6	3.9	61.6	4.0	642	1 cup	190
Others, baked, pork and molasses	125	70.0	5.8	3.0	2.0	19.2	.9	325	Baked, 1 cup	260
Others, baked, pork and tomato sauce	113	71.7	5.8	2.1	2.0	18.4	1.0	295	Baked, 1 cup	260
Lima, green, raw	128	66.5	7.5	.8	1.7	23.5	1.5	96	Green, raw, ½ cup	75
Lima, green, cooked	95	74.9	5.0	.4	1.4	18.3	2.0	152	Cooked, 1 cup	160
Lima, green, canned	71	80.9	3.8	.3	1.5	13.5	1.3	176	Canned, 1 cup	249
Lima, green, frozen	100	73.2	6.1	.2	1.5	19.0	1.7	75	Frozen, ½ cup	75
Lima, dry	333	12.6	20.7	1.3	3.8	61.6	4.3	610	Dry, 1 cup	183
Snap, green, raw	35	88.9	2.4	.2	.8	7.7	1.4	26	Raw, ¼ cup	75
Snap, green, cooked	22	92.5	1.4	.2	1.2	4.7	.5	27	Cooked, 1 cup	125
Snap, green, canned	18	93.5	1.0	.1	1.2	4.2	.6	27	Canned, 1 cup	125
Snap, green, frozen	27	91.6	1.7	.1	.5	6.2	1.1	20	Frozen, ¼ cup	75
Broccoli, raw	29	89.9	3.3	.2	1.1	5.5	1.3	25	Raw, 1 cup	120
Broccoli, cooked	29	89.9	3.3	.2	1.1	5.5	1.3	44	Cooked, 1 cup	150
Broccoli, frozen	30	90.2	3.4	.3	.8	5.3	1.1	36	Frozen, 1 cup	120
Cauliflower, raw	25	91.7	2.4	.2	.8	4.9	.9	31	Raw, 1¼ cups	125
Cauliflower, cooked	25	91.7	2.4	.2	.8	4.9	.9	30	Cooked, 1 cup	120
Cauliflower, frozen	22	92.7	2.1	.2	.6	4.3	.9	27	Frozen, 1¼ cups	125
Corn, sweet, raw	92	73.9	3.7	1.2	.7	20.5	.8	92	1 ear, 8″ long	100
Corn, sweet, cooked	85	75.5	2.7	.7	.9	20.2	—	85	Cooked, 1 ear, 5″	140
Corn, sweet, canned	67	80.5	2.0	.5	.9	16.1	.8	140	Canned, 1 cup	116
Cucumbers, raw	12	96.1	.7	.1	.4	2.7	.5	6	6, ⅛″ slices	50
Eggplant, raw	24	92.7	1.1	.2	.5	5.5	.9	60	2 slices	250
Lentils, dry split	339	12.2	24.0	1.2	2.2	60.4	1.7	204	¼ cup	60

FOOD COMPOSITION (continued)
CONSTITUENTS OF 100 g OF EDIBLE PORTION

Name	PROXIMATE COMPOSITION							AVERAGE PORTION		
	Cal-ories	Water, g	Pro-tein, g	Fat, g	Ash, g	Total Carbohy-drates, g	Crude Fiber, g	Total Calories	Measure	Weight in grams
Mushrooms, raw	16	91.1	2.4	.3	1.1	4.0	.9	8	½ cup, diced	50
Mushrooms, canned	11	93.0	1.4	.2	1.0	3.7	—	28	Canned, 1 cup	244
Okra, cooked	32	89.8	1.8	.2	.8	7.4	1.0	28	Cooked, 8 pods	85
Peas, green, raw	98	74.3	6.7	.4	.9	17.7	2.2	74	½ cup	75
Peas, green, cooked	70	81.7	4.9	.4	.9	12.1	2.2	111	Cooked, 1 cup	60
Peas, green, canned	68	82.3	3.4	.4	1.0	12.9	1.4	145	Canned, 1 cup	60
Peas, green, frozen	83	80.3	5.7	.4	.8	12.9	1.8	124	Frozen, 1 cup	150
Peas, dry, split	344	10.0	24.5	1.0	2.8	61.7	1.2	689	Dry, split, 1 cup	200
Peppers, green, raw	25	92.4	1.2	.2	.5	5.7	1.4	16	1 medium	76
Pumpkin, raw	31	90.5	1.2	.2	.8	7.3	1.3	37	Raw, ¾ cup	120
Pumpkin, canned	33	90.2	1.0	.3	.6	7.9	1.2	76	Canned, 1 cup	228
Soybeans, dry	331	7.5	34.9	18.1	4.7	34.8	5.0	695	Dry, 1 cup	210
Soybean flour, med. fat	264	9	42.5	6.5	4.8	37.2	2.6	232	1 cup	88
Soybean sprouts, raw	46	86.3	6.2	1.4	.8	5.3	.8	50	Raw, 1 cup	107
Squash, summer, raw	16	95.0	.6	.1	.4	3.9	.5	40	1¾ cups, diced	250
Squash, summer, frozen	21	93.4	1.4	.1	.4	4.7	.6	44	Cooked, diced, 1 cup	210
Squash, winter, raw	38	88.6	1.5	.3	.8	8.8	1.4	95	1¾ cups, diced	250
Squash, winter, cooked	47	85.7	1.9	.4	1.0	11.0	1.8	97	Mashed, 1 cup	205
Squash, winter, frozen	33	89.2	1.2	.4	.51	8.8	1.2	82	1¾ cups, diced	250
Succotash, frozen	97	66.3	4.5	.4	.8	21.4	.9	205	¾ cup, cooked	210
Tomatoes, raw	20	94.1	1.0	.3	.6	4.0	.6	30	1 med., 2 × 2½"	150
Tomatoes, canned	19	94.2	1.0	.2	.7	3.9	.4	46	Canned, 1 cup	242
Tomato ketchup	98	69.5	2.0	.4	3.6	24.5	.4	17	1 tbsp	17
Tomato puree, canned	36	89.2	1.8	.5	1.3	7.2	.4	90	1 cup	249
MISCELLANEOUS										
Beer (4% alcohol)	20–48	90.2	.6	0	.2	4.4	—	72–173	12 oz	360
Coffee, black	4	99	.2	0	—	.7	0	9	1 cup	230
Cola beverages	46	88	—	—	—	12	—	83	6 oz	180
Ginger ale	35	91	—	—	—	9	—	63	6 oz	180
Popcorn	386	4.0	12.7	5.0	1.6	76.7	2.2	54	1 cup, popped	14
Potato chips	544	3.1	6.7	37.1	4.0	49.1	1.1	108	10 medium, 2"	20
Yeast, bakers', compressed	86	70.9	10.6	.4	2.4	13.0	.3	24	1 oz	28
Yeast, brewers', dry	273	7.0	36.9	1.6	7.9	37.4	.8	22	1 tbsp	8

Index

Steven R. Peikin, M.D., was born in Philadelphia, where he attended Temple University and Jefferson Medical College of Thomas Jefferson University. After medical school he trained at the University of California, San Francisco, the National Institutes of Health, and Massachusetts General Hospital, and became board certified in internal medicine and gastroenterology. He is presently associate professor of medicine and pharmacology at Jefferson Medical College of Thomas Jefferson University, Director of the Jefferson Nutrition Program, and nutritional consultant for the Philadelphia Eagles football team. Dr. Peikin is an honorary fellow of the University of Liverpool, United Kingdom. He is internationally known for his research on gastrointestinal hormones and the control of food intake.

Dr. Peikin lives with his sons, Scott and Jeffrey, and wife, Lori Snodgrass, in suburban Philadelphia.

Gloria Kaufer Greene is the author of *The Jewish Holiday Cookbook: An International Collection of Recipes and Customs* (Times Books, 1985) and coauthor of *Don't Tell 'Em It's Good for 'Em* (Times Books, 1984) and *Eat Your Vegetables!* (Times Books, 1985).

During her career as a food journalist, Ms. Greene has written over 400 articles on cooking and nutrition. Since 1980, she has been food editor of the *Baltimore Jewish Times.* Her work has appeared in numerous publications, including the *Washington Post, Food and Wine, Family Circle, Hadassah Magazine, McCall's, Baltimore Magazine,* and *Mademoiselle.* She is a member of the International Association of Cooking Professionals.

Ms. Greene also teaches cooking classes and lectures widely on food-related subjects. She lives in Columbia, Maryland, with her husband, Geoffrey E. Greene, and their three sons, Dylan, Trevor and Jared.